Pharmacy Technician Certification

Quick-Study Guide

Second Edition

NOTICE

The authors and publisher have made a conscientious effort to ensure that the information in this study guide is accurate and in accord with accepted standards at the time of publication. However, the information should be used solely for course work and preparation for the examination given by the Pharmacy Technician Certification Board. In no event should the information contained herein be used in connection with the actual services to be performed by pharmacy technicians.

This book is in no way authorized by or sponsored by the Pharmacy Technician Certification Board, Inc.

Pharmacy Technician Certification

Quick-Study Guide

Second Edition

Susan Moss Marks, R.Ph.
Educational Services Consultant
Pharmacist and Technician Programs
Phoenix, Arizona

William A. Hopkins, Jr., Pharm.D.
President
Clinical Pharmacy Consultants of North Georgia
Atlanta, Georgia

American Pharmaceutical Association
Washington, D.C.

APhA

Editor: Julian I. Graubart
Managing Editor: Melanie Segala
Compositor: Anita Klein
Cover Designer: Mary Margaret Hiller

Published by the American Pharmaceutical Association,
2215 Constitution Avenue, N.W., Washington, DC 20037-2985
(http://www.aphanet.org)

Library of Congress Cataloging-in-Publication Data

Marks, Susan Moss.
Pharmacy technician certification: quick-study guide/Susan Moss Marks, Willaim A. Hopkins Jr.—2nd ed.
p. ; cm.
Includes bibliographical references.
ISBN 1-58212-000-5
1. Pharmacy technicians—Examinations, questions, etc. 2. Pharmacy technicians—Outlines, syllabi, etc. I. Hopkins, William A. (William Alexander), 1947.
II. Title.
[DNLM: 1. Pharmacy—Examination Questions. 2. Pharmacy—Outlines. 3. Pharmacists' Aides—Examination Questions. 4. Pharmacists' Aides—Outlines. QV 18.2 M346p 1999]
RS122.95.M37 1999
615'.1'076
99-050354

Printed in Canada

Contents

Foreword

The American Pharmaceutical Association (APhA) created the *Pharmacy Technician Certification Quick-Study Guide* in 1995 as part of its official policy in support of an expanding, knowledgeable corps of pharmacy technicians. The second edition of the *Quick-Study Guide,* like the first, is designed to serve as a resource for pharmacy technicians as they prepare for the national Pharmacy Technician Certification Examination and for technician educators and employers and state pharmacy organizations as they develop exam review courses. Today, the "Purple Book" is recognized by pharmacists and pharmacy technicians nationwide as a great resource for both these purposes.

The Pharmacy Technician Certification Board (PTCB) was established in January 1995 through a year-long effort by the founding organizations—APhA, American Society of Health-System Pharmacists, Illinois Council of Health-System Pharmacists (formerly the Illinois Council of Hospital Pharmacists), and Michigan Pharmacists Association—to create one consolidated, voluntary national certification program for pharmacy technicians.

APhA also served as a sponsor of the Scope of Pharmacy Practice Project, a national study of pharmacy practice. The project delineated functions and responsibilities of pharmacists and pharmacy technicians. Functions that relate to the work of technicians are described in the PTCB *Candidate Handbook* content outline, the basis for this publication. This content outline is new, having been updated in August of 1999.

The *Quick-Study Guide* specifically addresses the three broad function areas described in the content outline:

1. Assisting the pharmacist in serving patients—64% of the examination;
2. Maintaining medication and inventory control systems—25% of the examination; and
3. Participating in the administration and management of pharmacy practice—11% of the examination.

The *Quick-Study Guide* also includes a special fourth section on pharmaceutical calculations, which has been expanded considerably in this edition. An all new Chapter 12, Practice Questions, offers 67 questions to help readers assess their understanding of the material covered in the rest of the book.

This small volume is not a comprehensive review of required knowledge, nor is it a practice exam book. It is designed to be used alone as a refresher course or in conjunction with more detailed publications now on the market.

Several such references can help technicians and their educators or employers review important information in preparation for the exam, and a few contain sample questions and self-tests. These publications are listed in Appendix C.

Since we published the first edition of *Pharmacy Technician Certification Quick-Study Guide,* APhA has initiated a category of pharmacy technician membership, and at this writing nearly 3,000 pharmacy technicians have joined. We invite all pharmacy technicians to consider membership in APhA. For membership information, phone us toll free at (800) 237-2742 and ask for Member Services; write to us at APhA, Membership Department, 2215 Constitution Avenue, N.W., Washington, DC 20037; or check us out on the World Wide Web (http://www.aphanet.org).

John A. Gans, Pharm.D.
Executive Vice President
American Pharmaceutical Association

Section I

Assisting the Pharmacist in Serving Patients

Includes activities related to prescription dispensing and medication distribution, including:

- receiving and processing prescriptions and medication orders
- obtaining and entering information onto the patient profile
- collecting data to help the pharmacist monitor patient outcomes
- preparing sterile products

Chapter One

Receiving Prescriptions and Medication Orders

I. Key Terms and Concepts

A. Prescriptions

1. A prescription is an order for the preparation and administration of a drug or nondrug remedy issued by a licensed medical practitioner who is authorized by state law to prescribe. Prescriptions may be presented to the pharmacy in written form or via telephone, fax, or computer, depending on individual state laws. Prescribers may include physicians, dentists, veterinarians, nurse practitioners, and physician assistants. Prescriptions are usually filled in an outpatient pharmacy for use by the patient on an ambulatory basis.

B. Medication orders

1. A medication order, like a prescription, is a written order for the preparation and administration of medication, issued by a licensed medical practitioner who is authorized to prescribe. Medication orders are intended for patients in an inpatient (institutional) setting.

C. Trade/proprietary drug name

1. The terms *trade* and *proprietary* refer to the manufacturer's brand name (protected by trademark) for a particular drug.

D. Generic/nonproprietary drug name

1. The terms *generic* and *nonproprietary* refer to a drug name not protected by a trademark, usually descriptive of its chemical structure.

II. Understanding Prescriptions and Medication Orders

A. Prescriptions should contain the following information:

1. Patient information
    a. The prescription order should include the patient's name, age, address, and telephone number.
2. Date
    a. The date the prescriber wrote the prescription order.
3. Name of the product
    a. The drug name may be written as either the generic or trade name.
4. Strength of the product
    a. The strength should always be included to avoid misinterpretation, but may not be included if only one strength is commercially available, or if otherwise inappropriate (e.g., devices). Strength may also be excluded in products that consist of a combination of two or more drugs for which only one drug–drug concentration ratio is commercially available.
5. Dosage form
    a. The dosage form may not be included if only one dosage form is commercially available. See Appendix A for a list of common dosage forms.
6. Quantity of medication to be dispensed
    a. The number of units or dosage forms (e.g., tablets, ounces, grams) to be dispensed. May not be included if the quantity to be dispensed can be calculated from the physician's directions and duration of therapy. May also be written as q.s. *(a sufficient quantity)* or q.s. ad *(a sufficient quantity to make)*.
7. Directions for preparation
    a. Instructions to the pharmacist for compounding or preparing a product may be included. See Appendix B for terminology and abbreviations frequently used for this purpose.
8. Directions for labeling
    a. Prescriber's instructions to the pharmacist on what information should be included on the prescription label.

9. Directions for the patient to be included on the prescription label
    a. Instructions for the patient on how to use the medication properly. Appendix B lists terminology and abbreviations frequently used.
        (1) Route of administration. See Appendix A for a list of drug administration routes.
        (2) Dosage and dosage schedule. The quantity of medication to be taken by the patient and the schedule (frequency and/or time) of administration.
10. Refill information
    a. The prescriber's instructions for the number of refills that may be dispensed from the prescription order. If no information is provided, no refills are authorized. A prescriber may also write "no refills" or "NR" on the prescription order.
11. Prescriber information
    a. Prescriber name, address, and telephone number
    b. Prescriber's Drug Enforcement Administration (DEA) number
    c. Prescriber's signature (unless the prescription is received by telephone)

B. Medication orders
1. Patient information
    a. While every medication order may not include in-depth patient information (diagnosis, concurrent therapies, etc.), the patient profile should contain this information as transcribed from previous orders. Medication orders typically include the following information:
        (1) Patient's name, birth date, room number, identification number
        (2) Indication for use of the medication (why the drug is being ordered)
        (3) Allergies or other information necessary to process the medication order
2. Date the medication order was written

3. Time of day that the medication order was written
    a. Time is an important factor in the institutional setting where patients are cared for on a 24-hour basis.
4. Name of the product
    a. Generic and/or trade name of the product
5. Strength of the product
    a. The strength should always be included to avoid misinterpretation, but may not be included if only one strength is commercially available, or if otherwise inappropriate (e.g., devices). Strength may also be excluded in products that consist of a combination of two or more drugs for which only one drug:drug concentration ratio is commercially available.
6. Dosage form
    a. The dosage form may not be included if only one dosage form is commercially available. See Appendix A for a list of common dosage forms.
7. Prescriber information
    a. Name and signature of the prescriber. The prescriber is usually the patient's primary physician, but may be another attending physician or resident. The signature of the prescriber is not required when the order is received verbally, either by telephone or through another authorized health care professional. In these cases, the name or initial of the recipient (e.g., attending registered nurse or pharmacist) must be included on the medication order.
8. Directions for preparation
    a. Instructions to the pharmacist for compounding or preparing a product may be included. See Appendix B for terminology and abbreviations frequently used for this purpose.
9. Directions for administration
    a. Instructions for the nurse or other health care provider on how to administer the medication properly.
        (1) Route of administration. See Appendix A for a list of drug administration routes.

(2) Dosage and dosage schedule. The quantity of medication to be taken and the schedule (frequency and/or time) of administration.

b. Duration of therapy. Instructions describing how long the patient should receive the medication.

c. Other instructions for administration. This may include detailed information on administration and scheduling of the drug such as start date for medication use, tapering dosages, administration times related to laboratory tests, etc.

III. Receiving New Prescriptions and Medication Orders

A. Accepting new prescriptions/medication orders from patient/patient's representative, prescriber, or other health care professionals. Performing this function requires the technician to be knowledgeable about the information required on prescriptions and medication orders.

1. Written orders

a. Ambulatory/outpatient setting

(1) Prescriptions may be presented to the pharmacy in various ways. In the outpatient setting, new prescriptions are typically brought to the pharmacy in written form by the patient or patient's representative. Depending on state laws, the prescriber may also send written prescription orders via fax.

b. Institutional/inpatient setting

(1) In the institutional setting, a written medication order may be presented to the pharmacy department by a physician, nurse, other health care professional or messenger; transmitted electronically through an in-house computer system; or sent to the pharmacy via a pneumatic tube system.

2. Electronic prescriptions/medication orders

a. Fax and computer-generated prescriptions/medication orders

(1) Fax and computer-generated orders are electronic versions of written orders and should be received and assessed in the same manner.

3. Telephone orders

   a. Verbal orders for medications (whether received by telephone or in person) may be accepted only by a licensed pharmacist or, in some states, by a supervised pharmacy intern. In the institutional setting, a registered nurse may also receive and transcribe telephone orders from the prescriber.

IV. Receiving Prescription Refill and Transfer Requests

A. Accepting refill requests from patient/patient's representative or prescriber

   1. Receiving refill requests requires the technician to be knowledgeable about what information is required to process refills and how to obtain appropriate authorization for refills if necessary.

B. Accepting refill requests electronically

   1. Telephone orders

      a. The following information should be obtained when receiving oral requests for refills from patients, patients' representatives, or prescribers:

         (1) Patient name and telephone number

         (2) Prescription number

         (3) Drug name, strength, and quantity

         (4) Prescriber information

         (5) Reimbursement mechanisms/third-party-payer information

   2. Fax and computer-generated refill requests

      a. The information listed above also should be included in fax requests for refills. The prescriber must be contacted if more information is needed.

C. Contacting prescribers for clarification/authorization of prescription or medication order refills

   1. At the direction of the supervising pharmacist, technicians may be responsible for calling prescribers to obtain authorization for prescription refills or to renew medication orders that have expired. The following information should be provided to the prescriber or the prescriber's representative:

a. Pharmacy's name and telephone number

b. Patient's name

c. Drug name, strength, and quantity

d. Date of last refill

e. Prescription directions

f. Description of information that needs to be clarified, confirmed, or authorized

D. Transferring and accepting transfers of prescription or medication orders

1. At the direction of the supervising pharmacist, technicians may be responsible for transferring prescriptions to another pharmacy or receiving prescriptions transferred by another pharmacy. The following information should be provided to the pharmacy receiving the transfer, and requested by the technician or pharmacist accepting a transferred prescription:

a. Pharmacy's name and telephone number

b. Patient's name and telephone number

c. Drug name, strength, quantity, and instructions for use

d. Date of original prescription

e. Date of last refill

f. Doctor's name and telephone number

g. Names of technicians or pharmacists sending and receiving the transferred prescription

h. Original prescription number

V. Assessing Prescription/Medication Orders

A. Assessing the order for accuracy and completeness requires the technician to understand the information being presented and to ask appropriate questions when necessary. Evaluating the prescription or medication order should include checking the accuracy and completeness of the following:

1. Patient information. Using the criteria described above, ascertain that appropriate patient information is included on the prescription/medication order.

a. Prescriptions

(1) Patient's name, age, address, known allergies

b. Medication orders

(1) Patient's name, birth date, room number, identification number, allergies, indications, and any other pertinent information necessary for processing the medication order. Other relevant patient information (e.g., diagnosis) may be verified by checking the patient profile.

2. Drug or product information

a. Consistency with products currently available on the market. Verify that the product or drug name, strength, and dosage form are written in a manner consistent with commercially available products. This requires knowledge of available products, prescription medications, dosage forms, strengths, etc.

3. Authenticity

a. Assess whether the prescription/medication order appears to be legitimate (e.g., prescriber's signature is authentic).

4. Legality

a. Assess whether the prescription/medication order is legal. This includes verifying that the order is in compliance with federal and state laws, etc.

5. Reimbursement eligibility

a. Includes assessing whether the patient is covered by the appropriate insurance or third-party payer and that the drug (and the quantity of drug prescribed) is eligible for reimbursement based on the policies of the payer. Confirm that the pharmacy accepts the patient's insurance carrier.

VI. Chapter Summary

A. As front-line health care practitioners, pharmacy technicians must understand all aspects of receiving prescription and medication orders.

B. Technicians should be familiar with information required on prescription and medication orders. They must also know how to accept new orders, refill requests and transfers from health care professionals, and be able to assess orders for clarity, completeness, accuracy, authenticity, and legality.

VII. Questions for Discussion

A. Discuss various differences between prescription orders and medication orders (information requirements, intent, etc.).

B. What action should you take when a patient requests a refill of a prescription that does not have refills authorized?

C. What factors should the technician consider when evaluating the authenticity of a prescription/medication order?

D. What factors should the technician consider when evaluating the accuracy and completeness of a prescription/medication order?

E. Why is the time of day that a medication order is written important in the institutional setting? Discuss examples of problems that could occur when time is not included on the order.

F. What action should you take when the pharmacy receives a prescription faxed from a patient or a patient's representative?

VIII. Sample Questions

A. What information is required on prescription orders but not required on medication orders?

1. Patient information
2. Date
3. Dosage form
4. Quantity to be dispensed
5. Directions for preparation

B. Prescriptions and medication orders must contain which of the following:

1. Generic name of the drug
2. Trade name of the drug
3. Dosage form
4. Either 1 or 2
5. All of the above answers are correct

C. True or false?

1. When there is only one brand/trade name for a medication (no generic equivalent), the trade name must appear on the prescription/medication order.
2. Telephone orders for new prescriptions may only be received by a registered pharmacist or, in some states, by a supervised pharmacy intern, but technicians may telephone prescribers for the authorization of refills.
3. If the prescriber writes "no refills" or "NR" on the prescription order, the prescription may never be refilled.

D. Which of the following are commercially available products?

1. Diazepam 15 mg capsules
2. Clarithromycin 500 mg tablets
3. Benazepril hydrochloride 30 mg tablets
4. Fluconazole 400 mg injection
5. Idarubicin 10 mg capsules
6. Cefadroxil 125 mg/5 ml oral solution
7. Albuterol sulfate 2 mg/5 ml oral syrup
8. Cyclobenzaprine 100 mg tablets
9. Prednisone 50 mg tablets
10. Indomethacin 50 mg suppositories
11. Nortriptyline 20 mg capsules
12. Clindamycin 300 mg tablets
13. Felodipine 10 mg tablets
14. Etodolac 300 mg tablets
15. Timolol maleate 0.25% solution
16. Digoxin 5 mg tablet
17. Phenobarbital 15 mg tablet

E. Transcribe the following abbreviated instructions into readable directions as they should appear on a prescription label. Include leading verbs (take, inject, etc.).

1. ii tab p.o. q.i.d.
2. i cap a.c. & h.s.
3. 5 mg. IM q 3–4 h p.r.n. nausea
4. i gtt. o.d. q 12 h
5. ii–iii gtt. a.u. t.i.d.
6. i gtt. a.u. b.i.d.

F. Which of the following describes routes of drug administration?

1. Suppository
2. Injection
3. Otic
4. Answers 1. and 2. are correct
5. All of the above answers are correct

G. What instruction might be included on the prescription label for a suspension?

1. Shake well
2. Keep refrigerated
3. Apply to affected areas three times daily
4. Answers 1. and 2. are correct
5. All of the above answers are correct

Answers to sample questions appear on page 109.

Chapter Two

Patient Information/ Profile Systems

I. Key Terms and Concepts

A. Patient profile

1. A record containing information pertaining to a specific patient including demographic information, medical history, medication use chronology, allergies, and chronic illnesses. Patient profiles may be manual (printed information in files) or computerized.

B. Diagnosis

1. The identified disease or health condition determined by the prescriber through assessment of the patient's signs and symptoms. Also refers to the art or act of identifying a disease from its signs and symptoms.

C. Psychosocial factors

1. Involving both psychological and social aspects; relating social conditions to mental health.

D. Socioeconomic factors

1. Of, relating to, or involving a combination of social and economic factors.

E. Desired therapeutic outcome

1. The desired health result of drug therapy. The outcome may be an end result (e.g., complete cure of the disease), a goal related to incurable but controllable disease states (e.g., lowering and maintaining blood pressure to an acceptable level in a hypertensive patient), or a general goal of therapy (e.g., an appropriate level of sedation prior to surgery).

II. Assisting the Pharmacist in Obtaining Patient Information to be Entered in the Patient Profile

A. Obtaining patient information

1. At the direction of the pharmacist, technicians may be required to ask patient/patient's representative, prescriber, or other health professional for certain types of information. This information, while important to the patient's use of a specific drug or drug regimen, is also used to create or update the patient profile. Technicians should possess good communication skills and be knowledgeable about appropriate patient interviewing techniques.

B. Patient profiles

1. Patient profiles may be manual or computerized records. The following information may be included in a patient profile:

    a. Patient information

        (1) Ambulatory/outpatient setting

            (a) Patient's name, birth date, address, telephone number, pertinent insurance reimbursement information

        (2) Institutional/inpatient setting

            (a) Patient's name, birth date, address, height, weight, identification number, room number, primary physician

2. Diagnosis
3. Desired therapeutic outcome
4. Medication use

    a. The patient's medication history and current medication use (including nonprescription drugs) is critical to assessing the appropriateness of therapy. This information may be used to detect potential drug interactions, possible allergies, medication duplication, and other potential problems. The outpatient profile should include a chronology of medication refills.

5. Allergies

    a. The patient's history of allergies may predict potential allergies to similar drugs.

6. Adverse reactions
   a. The patient's history of adverse reactions may help predict potential adverse reactions to similar drugs.
7. Medical history
   a. This includes a chronology of past and current medical conditions.
8. Psychosocial history
   a. This is important because of its potential influence on patient compliance, drug misuse, drug abuse, and other factors. In some cases, the pharmacist may need to give the patient additional instructions or counseling.
9. Patient characteristics/special considerations
   a. These include characteristics that require special attention when processing the patient's prescriptions. Addressing these factors will help prevent potential problems (e.g., compliance, drug misuse). Patients with limitations may require special labeling, packaging, auxiliary materials (e.g., instructions written in large print or in another language), or counseling by the pharmacist. Examples include:
      (1) Physical characteristics
         (a) Visual impairment
         (b) Hearing impairment
         (c) Other physical disability
      (2) Sociological characteristics
         (a) Foreign language
         (b) Cultural or religious beliefs
10. Socioeconomic history
11. Reimbursement mechanisms and third-party-payer information
   a. This function includes questioning the patient/patient's representative about the payment method, and assessing the eligibility of the patient (and the prescribed product) for reimbursement from the patient's third-party payer.

C. Collecting data to monitor patient outcomes
   1. At the direction of the pharmacist, technicians may collect data that will help the pharmacist monitor patient outcomes. Tests may include:

a. Blood pressure measurements in those with pre-existing or suspected hypertension.

b. Glucose (blood sugar) levels in diabetics, those suspected of having diabetes, or pregnant women who have had problems with elevated glucose levels.

c. Blood lipid analysis (cholesterol, low-density lipoproteins, [LDL], high-density lipoproteins [HDL], etc.).

III. Entering Patient Information in the Patient Profile

A. New patients

1. Patient profiles are generated for every patient receiving medications from the pharmacy department. Working with the pharmacist, technicians may be asked to create a profile for each new patient who receives a prescription or medication order from the pharmacy.

B. Patients with existing profiles

1. Updating the medical record/patient profile

a. Because the patient's health status and/or response to medications may change, patient profiles must be updated as often as necessary. The patient/patient's representative may not automatically volunteer this information; therefore, at the direction of the pharmacist, technicians may interview patients about possible changes in their health condition or medication use. Any of the items listed in the patient profile may need to be updated. Changes in patient information other than demographics (e.g., address) should be brought to the pharmacist's attention immediately so that the patient can be counseled appropriately. The most common changes include:

(1) Patient information. Ask the patient/patient's representative whether this information is correct and current.

(2) Diagnosis or desired therapeutic outcome. Has anything changed regarding the patient's

disease or condition? Are there any new problems?

(3) Medication use. Is the patient still using the medications listed in the patient profile? Have any new prescription or nonprescription medications been added to the regimen?

(4) Allergies. Has the patient experienced allergic symptoms that may be related to current drug therapy?

(5) Adverse reactions. Has the patient experienced adverse reactions that may be related to current drug therapy?

(6) Reimbursement mechanisms and third-party-payer information. Is this information correct and current?

(7) Medication duplication. When updating the patient profile, it is important to be aware of the possibility of medication duplication. If discovered, the pharmacist should be notified immediately.

(8) Drug interactions. Be aware of the potential for drug interactions. Prescription drugs may interact with other prescription drugs, nonprescription drugs, food, and some laboratory tests.

IV. Chapter Summary

A. Developing and maintaining patient profile systems is a primary responsibility of technicians in both inpatient and outpatient settings.

B. Technicians must be knowledgeable about the patient information that is included in profiles and important changes that require special attention by the pharmacist.

C. Pharmacy technicians may assist the pharmacist in obtaining patient information by conducting interviews with patients or their representatives, and with health care professionals. To do this effectively, technicians must possess good communication skills and be proficient in various interviewing techniques. Obtaining information about a patient's diagnosis, desired therapeutic outcome, medication use, allergies, and other pertinent data is essential to the provision of complete pharmaceutical care.

D. Performing tests for elevated blood pressure, glucose, and cholesterol helps the pharmacist monitor the patient's therapeutic outcome. The technician can play a key role in this type of monitoring.

V. Questions for Discussion

A. Accepting new prescriptions/medication orders may require the technician to interview the patient/patient's representative about certain types of information.

1. What types of questions should be asked of a new patient?
2. What questions should be asked of a patient who has an existing patient profile?

B. Describe examples of psychosocial factors that may be important to consider when obtaining patient information for the patient profile.

C. How do a patient's psychosocial history and socioeconomic status affect the patient's ability to adhere to a prescribed therapeutic regimen?

D. Discuss ways the pharmacy technician can increase compliance in patients with physical disabilities.

E. Describe examples of medication and/or medication class duplication.

F. Discuss the importance of good communication skills in patient interviewing. What communication skills are most important?

G. Describe symptoms associated with an allergic reaction.

VI. Sample Questions

A. True or false?

1. Nonprescription drugs should not be included in the patient profile.
2. Patient profiles should be created for every patient for whom a prescription/medication order is presented to the pharmacy.
3. Changes in patient information other than demographics should be brought to the attention of the supervising pharmacist.
4. Obtaining patient information to enter in the patient profile is almost never performed by the pharmacy technician.

B. When updating the patient profile, the technician may ask about all of the following types of information except

1. Patient's use of over-the-counter medications
2. Changes in insurance coverage
3. Other prescriptions that the patient is receiving that are being provided by the physician or other pharmacies
4. Laboratory tests the patient is scheduled to undergo
5. All of the above types of information are important to be included in the patient profile

Answers to sample questions appear on page 109.

Chapter Three

Processing Prescriptions and Medication Orders

I. Key Terms and Concepts

A. Pharmacology

1. The science that deals with the origin, nature, chemistry, effects, and uses of drugs

B. Compounding

1. The act or process of combining two or more drug products or chemicals into a single preparation

C. Controlled substances

1. Drugs that are regulated under the Controlled Substances Act, a federal law enacted in 1970. It regulates the prescribing and dispensing of drugs of abuse, according to five schedules (designated I, II, III, IV, and V) based on their abuse potential, medical acceptance, and ability to produce dependence (addiction). The law also established a regulatory system for the manufacture, storage, and transport of the drugs in each schedule. Drugs covered by this Act include opium and its derivatives, opiates, hallucinogens, depressants, stimulants, and anabolic steroids.

D. Sterile

1. Aseptic; free from microorganisms and not producing microorganisms; containing no bacterial and viral contaminants.

E. I.V. Admixtures

1. Intravenous solutions compounded with two or more ingredients (i.e., one or more additives mixed with the primary intravenous solution).

F. Laminar Airflow Hood

1. Equipment used for the preparation of sterile products that provides filtered air, flowing horizontally or vertically, to prevent contamination by microorganisms. Horizontal airflow hoods are generally used in the preparation of most products. Vertical airflow hoods are used for the preparation of cytotoxic drugs to protect the operator from exposure to these agents.

G. Cytotoxic Agents/Cytotoxins

1. An agent that has a specific toxic action upon cells of susceptible organs. Cytotoxic agents are commonly used to treat many forms of cancer (neoplasms).

H. Antineoplastic Agents

1. An agent that is used to treat neoplasms (cancers).

II. Understanding Drug Actions and Uses

A. Pharmacology and drug classifications

1. Technicians should be knowledgeable about drug actions and pharmacological classifications. Some of the publications listed in Appendix C may be useful in reviewing pharmacology.

III. Entering Prescription or Medication Order Information onto the Patient Profile

A. Entering new prescription/medication information in an existing patient profile or creating a new patient profile is usually the first step in processing prescriptions/medication orders. Strict attention to detail when performing this function is critical because entry errors can directly affect patient safety. This function may also provide input into other systems. For example, entering the prescription/medication order into a computerized patient profile may simultaneously generate a prescription label, update the drug inventory record, create an entry into a "want book" or other ordering system, and update or change information in other databases. Steps to follow when entering new prescription/medication information include:

1. Verify the patient's name and/or identification number. If the patient already has an existing profile, confirm that the patient information on the new order matches the patient information on the profile. If no patient profile is found, a new profile must be created. For a complete discussion about information included in patient profiles, see Chapter Two.
2. Compare the new order with the patient profile. Look for medication duplication (the patient is already receiving the drug), drug class duplication (e.g., an order for the diuretic furosemide to be dispensed to a patient who is already receiving hydrochlorothiazide), or other possible problems. If problems are discovered, the pharmacist should be notified immediately before proceeding.
3. Enter the date, drug name, dosage form, quantity to be dispensed, directions for use, and number of refills, if any.
4. Enter the prescriber information and the initials of the technician and supervising pharmacist dispensing the medication (how this information is entered may vary, depending on the pharmacy).
5. Enter the reimbursement mechanism or third-party-payer information.
6. Enter other information as required by the pharmacy's policies and procedures.

IV. Selecting Appropriate Product(s) to be Dispensed

A. Selecting the appropriate drug to be dispensed for a prescription or medication order

1. Prescriptions and medication orders should be filled from the original order to minimize errors. While filling the order, the technician must meticulously scrutinize the information that has been entered in the patient profile and on the prescription label, carefully comparing it with the original prescription/medication order.

B. Selecting the manufacturing source of the product(s) to be dispensed for a prescription or medication order. Prescriptions and medication orders may be written in two ways:

1. Generic terminology
    a. When a pharmaceutical manufacturer's patent expires for a proprietary drug, other companies may obtain approval from the Food and Drug Administration (FDA) to manufacture and market their own version of the drug. Because of individual policies and purchasing contracts, each pharmacy may have a preferred manufacturing source for different generic drugs. When a prescription or medication order is written in generic terminology, the selection of which product to dispense is usually dependent on which manufacturer is the preferred source for that particular drug. The preferred source may also differ depending on the drug (e.g., the preferred source for hydrochlorothiazide tablets may be the ABC Company's generic brand, while the XYZ Company's generic acetaminophen may be the preferred generic product).
2. Trade or brand name terminology
    a. Appropriate methods for processing prescriptions and medication orders written in trade name terminology are dependent on policies and procedures related to several factors including state laws, third-party payers, and individual pharmacies or institutions.
        (1) Institutions. The pharmacy and therapeutics committee is usually charged with developing policies related to the use of drug products within the institution and creating formularies based on these decisions. The formulary restricts which drugs a physician may prescribe, and gives the pharmacy department authority to substitute a generic equivalent for a trade name product if one is available. Therefore, when a medication order is written in trade name terminology, it is common practice for the order to be filled with the preferred generic equivalent. If no generic equivalent exists (and the drug is on the formulary), the order is filled with the trade name product.
        (2) Community and ambulatory pharmacies. Each pharmacy may have its own set of policies and procedures, in addition to preferred generics as

mentioned above. Most commonly, third-party payers dictate whether the prescription will be filled (some medications aren't covered) and how they will be filled (trade brand or generic). Most payers require generic substitution when available. If a generic equivalent is available, it is common practice for the technician or pharmacist to ask the patient or the patient's representative if he or she will accept a generic substitute. If the patient or patient's representative prefers the trade name version that is not approved by his or her particular health insurance company, the patient will usually have to pay the difference in price to the pharmacy.

C. Obtaining medications or devices from inventory. After determining the manufacturing source of the product(s) to be dispensed, obtain the medications or devices from inventory.

D. Calibrating equipment needed to prepare or compound the prescription or medication order. As an important quality control measure, equipment used for measuring or compounding prescriptions and medication orders should be calibrated regularly to ensure accuracy. Each pharmacy department has policies and procedures that describe calibration methods and schedules to follow to ensure that equipment is maintained on a routine basis.

V. Preparing and Dispensing Medications to Fill Prescriptions and Medication Orders

A. Dispensing finished dosage forms

1. This includes measuring or counting finished dosage forms according to instructions on the original prescription or medication order.

B. Calculations

1. At the direction of the pharmacist, the technician may assist in performing and/or verifying pharmaceutical calculations. A thorough discussion of calculations is presented in Section IV.

C. Preparing intravenous admixtures and other sterile products

1. Procedures for the preparation of intravenous admixtures and other sterile products can be found in a variety of sources. Some of the publications included in Appendix C may be useful in reviewing aseptic technique. See Section IV for calculations related to the preparation of intravenous solutions.

D. Compounding medications for dispensing according to prescription formula or instructions

1. At the direction of the pharmacist, technicians may be asked to assist in the compounding function. See Section IV for a discussion of calculations related to compounding preparations.

E. Recording preparation of medication in various dosage forms

1. Information describing how the prescription was prepared should be documented on the prescription or medication order and on the patient profile.

F. Recording preparation of controlled substances for dispensing

1. By law, controlled substances require a strict inventory control system, and special documentation is required to record the dispensing of controlled substances as both established dosage forms and as ingredients of compounded preparations. Inventory control records are usually organized according to drug name and dosage form (i.e., each product has its own record). The following information may be required for adequate documentation:

   a. Date the drug was removed from inventory

   b. Amount of drug that was removed from inventory

   c. How the drug was used (e.g., in the preparation of a cough syrup)

   d. Patient and auxiliary information

      (1) Ambulatory/outpatient setting

         (a) Patient name, prescription number, prescriber

      (2) Institutional/inpatient setting

         (a) Patient name, room number, identification number

      (3) Technician and pharmacist initials

      (4) Other information

VI. Preparing Intravenous (I.V.) Admixtures and Other Sterile Products

Technicians may help institutionalized patients, and sometimes outpatients, by preparing sterile intravenous fluids containing drugs, vitamins, or other nutrients.

A. Sterile/Aseptic Technique
Compounding intravenous solutions, other types of injections (I.M., S.Q., etc.), ophthalmic and otic products, and other preparations that will be instilled directly into the patient's body tissues (e.g., irrigation solutions) requires strict adherence to aseptic technique to prevent contamination by microorganisms.

1. Each institution and ambulatory pharmacy has written policies describing the proper use of aseptic technique. This type of compounding is usually done in a separate sterile compounding room or in a specially designated area in the pharmacy. Correct use of this technique involves proper attire, efficient hand washing, sterilization of the surface (horizontal or vertical laminar airflow hood), aseptic preparation of the sterile products, and maintaining the sterility of the compounding area.

a. Proper attire for sterile technique

(1) Proper attire for pharmacists and technicians preparing sterile products consists of a sterile gown, sterile gloves, a face mask to cover the nose and mouth, and a cap to contain and cover the hair.

b. Hand washing

(1) The first step technicians must take before preparing sterile products is hand washing. Hands must be cleaned thoroughly using chlorhexidine or another disinfectant.

c. Sterilization of the compounding surface

(1) The sterilizing agent may vary with each institution or pharmacy. Ethyl alcohol (ethanol) and isopropyl alcohol (isopropanol or "rubbing alcohol") are the most commonly used agents. Alcohol is poured in a thick layer on the hood surface, wiped down with sterile gauze from back to front, and left wet until it evaporates. Leaving the compounding surface wet allows enough time for the alcohol to kill microorganisms that may be on the surface.

d. Sterilization of the injection sites on the additive containers

(1) Similarly, the injection site on the additive vial is saturated with an alcohol preparation. The site is then wiped with sterile gauze to clean the area where the needle is inserted to inject, reconstitute and withdraw the additive.

e. Maintaining the sterility of materials used to prepare aseptic products.

(1) While preparing aseptic products, care must be taken to keep all surfaces and materials sterile and to assure that they don't come into contact with other surfaces that may not be sterile, or may be contaminated with other medications or substances.

f. Maintaining the sterility of the compounding area

(1) The sterile compounding room or area must be scrupulously and continually maintained to assure that all products are prepared in a completely aseptic environment. Mandatory periodic tests are conducted to assure that this area is maintained properly and is contamination-free.

B. Compounding Sterile Preparations

1. Additives

a. Many drugs are stored in the pharmacy as sterile powders that must be reconstituted. Using aseptic technique, an appropriate amount of diluent (most commonly normal saline) is injected into the vial, the container is shaken, and then left on the hood surface until every particle of the powder is dissolved and the resultant solution is clear. It is then withdrawn from the vial and injected into a larger volume sterile solution. In some instances, the medication is withdrawn and dispensed in a labeled syringe to be injected directly into the patient, or into another I.V. the patient is receiving. Drugs that are available as solutions do not require reconstitution and may be withdrawn and added to the larger volume solution immediately.

2. Preventing cross-contamination

   a. While aseptic technique prevents bacterial contamination, it also guards against cross-contamination between two or more drugs. This is important to prevent serious and potentially fatal allergic reactions. Using aseptic technique, the syringe used to dilute or withdraw one medication is never used to dilute or withdraw another drug. Similarly, materials used in the compounding of one drug must not touch containers or other materials used to prepare a different medication.

3. Antineoplastic chemotherapy agents

   a. Most sterile products are prepared in a *horizontal* laminar airflow hood that directs filtered air horizontally toward the operator or technician to protect against contamination by microorganisms. Some chemotherapeutic agents used to treat cancer (neoplasms) are cytotoxic, and can be hazardous to the operator. For this reason, these agents are prepared in a *vertical* laminar airflow hood which directs filtered air vertically (from top to bottom of the hood) to protect the operator from possible adverse effects that may occur from exposure to these agents.

VII. Packaging Preparations

A. Prescriptions

1. Prescription preparations are usually packaged according to the requirements of the specific drug and/or dosage form. Most preparations, regardless of dosage form are packaged and dispensed in containers that protect the drug from light, which can hasten the degradation of drug products.

B. Medication orders

1. Unit-dose packaging

   a. Unit-dose packaging is employed for most drugs dispensed in the institutional setting. When not commercially available, the pharmacy department may use special equipment to package "bulk" medications into unit-dose forms.

2. Multiple-dose packaging

   a. Drugs may be dispensed in "bulk" (more than a single dosage, sometimes several days' supply of medication). Multiple-dose packaging is most commonly used for drugs not commercially available in unit-dose packaging and not used by the hospital in sufficient quantity to make repackaging into unit-dose forms feasible. These products will require labeling consistent with the requirements of prescription labels.

      (1) Single-day (24-hour) supply. The pharmacy department may dispense a 24-hour supply of the drug in a labeled prescription vial. This is most commonly used for oral dosage forms.

      (2) Multiple-day supply. For some dosage forms, it is not reasonable to attempt repackaging into a single-day supply (e.g., creams, ointments not available in unit-dose packages).

3. Packaging of sterile products

   a. Sterile products intended for intravenous or intramuscular injection are usually prepared by adding medications or nutrients to a sterile solution in the final container that will be aseptically sealed and dispensed. Sometimes, transferring solutions through intravenous tubing to the final container is required. A few preparations must be filtered before dispensing. The technician should be proficient in these techniques and knowledgeable about the individual processes required for each medication.

VIII. Labeling Prescriptions and Medication Orders

A. Prescriptions. Prescriptions should be labeled with the following information:

   1. Name and address of pharmacy
   2. Date the prescription was filled
   3. Prescription number
   4. Drug name (generic or trade), strength, and quantity

5. Directions for patient (administration route, schedule, duration)
6. Patient's name
7. Prescriber's name
8. Expiration date
9. Number of refills (if authorized)
10. Lot number
11. Pharmacist's initials
12. Auxiliary labels providing additional information on storage, administration guidelines, cautions, etc.
13. Other information required by state or federal laws
    a. Controlled substances
        (1) Federal transfer label

B. Medication orders

1. Unit-dose medications should be labeled with the following information (commercially available unit-dose products are already labeled by the manufacturer with the appropriate information, although auxiliary labels may be needed for some drugs):
    a. Drug name and strength
    b. Lot number
    c. Expiration date
    d. Directions for administration if necessary (e.g., for intramuscular injection only)
    e. Auxiliary labels if necessary (storage, administration guidelines, cautions, etc.)
2. Multiple-dose packages should be labeled with the following information:
    a. Patient's name and room number
    b. Drug name, strength, quantity
    c. Directions for administration
    d. Lot number
    e. Expiration date
    f. Auxiliary labels if necessary (storage, administration guidelines, cautions, etc.)
3. Sterile products should be labeled with the same information required on multiple-dose packages (above).

IX. Verifying Dispensing and Labeling Accuracy

A. Performing intermediate checks during processing of the prescription/medication order

1. Performing intermediate checks is critical during the dispensing and labeling process. Technicians must pay careful attention to the specific details of the prescription/medication order, continually comparing the original order, label, patient profile, and the drug selected for accuracy.
2. The technician may also be called upon to verify the measurements, preparation, and/or packaging of medications produced by other technicians.

B. Pharmacist authorization

1. Authorization from the supervising pharmacist must be obtained and documented before prescriptions/ medication orders are dispensed.

X. Compiling Patient Information Materials

A. At the direction of the pharmacist, the technician may be responsible for collecting supplemental patient information materials (e.g., patient package inserts, computer-generated information, videos) to be dispensed with the prescription/ medication order.

XI. Delivering Medications to the Patient or the Patient's Representative

A. The technician should be familiar with the following functions related to the delivery of medications to patients. Specific policies and procedures governing these functions may vary, depending on the institution or pharmacy.

1. Storing medications prior to distribution
    a. The technician should be familiar with the pharmacy's policies regarding storage of medications prior to distribution and also be knowledgeable about which medications require special storage conditions (e.g., refrigeration).

2. Delivering medication to the patient or patient's representative
   a. Ambulatory/outpatient setting
      (1) In some states, technicians may be authorized to make the offer to counsel.
   b. Institutional/inpatient setting
      (1) Placing medication in the unit-dose cart
      (2) Delivering medication to the patient-care unit
3. Recording distribution of prescription medications
4. Recording distribution of controlled substances

XII. Determining Charges and Obtaining Compensation for Services

A. Calculating charges
   1. Charges for prescriptions and medication orders vary depending on a specific pharmacy department's policies and third-party reimbursement plans. A review of calculations related to pricing prescriptions is presented in Chapter Eleven.

B. Communicating with third-party payers to determine or verify coverage
   1. The technician may be responsible for contacting third-party payers to verify the patient's eligibility for coverage.
   2. The technician may be responsible for contacting third-party payers for prior approval of nonformulary drugs and supplies.

C. Obtaining compensation
   1. Ambulatory/outpatient setting
      a. Payment from the patient or patient's representative
         (1) In the ambulatory setting, the first step in obtaining compensation is through receipt of a payment or partial payment (copayment) from the patient or the patient's representative.
      b. Reimbursement from third-party payers
         (1) For patients covered by third-party plans, the second step in obtaining compensation is through contact with the specific company providing prescription benefit coverage for the patient. The technician may be responsible for

completing the appropriate paperwork (or computer-generated forms) to request reimbursement from various third-party payers.

2. Institutional/inpatient setting
   a. Patient billing
      (1) The pharmacy technician may be responsible for billing drug charges to the patient's account. The actual task of direct billing to patients and third-party payers is usually done by the institution's accounting department.

XIII. Providing Supplemental Information, as Indicated

A. The technician should ask all patients if counseling by a pharmacist is desired.

B. At the direction of the pharmacist, the technician may be responsible for giving the patient supplemental information materials along with the prescription/medication order. Types of patient information include:

1. Patient package inserts. FDA regulations require that patient package inserts (PPIs) be provided to patients receiving the following medications:
   a. Oral contraceptives
   b. Products containing estrogenic drugs
   c. Products containing progestational drugs
   d. Isotretinoin
   e. Intrauterine devices
   f. Isoproterenol inhalation products
2. Computer-generated information. As a component of many electronic prescription processing programs, computer-generated information is often routinely provided to patients.
3. Videos

XIV. Chapter Summary

A. Processing prescriptions and medication orders is a multifaceted operation requiring knowledge of many different aspects of pharmacy technician practice.

B. Preparation of sterile products and admixtures requires the technician to be proficient in the use of aseptic technique and knowledgeable about process requirements specific to each medication.

C. Strict attention to detail must be followed while performing multiple tasks, including reviewing the patient profile; selecting, preparing, packaging, and labeling the appropriate product to fill the order; verifying dispensing and labeling accuracy through intermediate checks; calculating patient charges and obtaining compensation from third party payers; and delivering the product and supplemental patient information to the patient or patient's representative.

XV. Questions for Discussion

A. Before the unit-dose system was developed, institutions typically dispensed a five-day supply of each regular medication, packaged and labeled in a prescription vial. Discuss the advantages and disadvantages of each system.

B. What factors should be considered when selecting the appropriate product to be dispensed for a prescription/ medication order?

C. Describe various types of packaging and discuss the advantages and disadvantages of each.

D. Describe the use of aseptic technique and processes used to prepare sterile products.

XVI. Sample Questions

A. True or false?

1. In the outpatient setting, pharmacists must authorize all prescription orders before the medications are dispensed to the patient; but in the institutional setting, pharmacist authorization is not required if the technician gives the drug directly to a registered nurse because nurses have the same authority.

2. In the institutional setting, multiple-dose packaging is preferred for certain oral dosage forms.
3. A supervising pharmacist must continually observe a technician preparing sterile products.

B. Unit-dose medications should be labeled with all of the following information except:

1. Lot number
2. Prescriber's name
3. Expiration date
4. Name of medication
5. Strength of medication

C. All of the following medications require patient package inserts to be dispensed with the prescription except:

1. Premarin®
2. Brevicon®
3. Ogen®
4. Accutane®
5. Vagitrol®

D. When selecting the appropriate product to fill a prescription/medication order, confusion caused by similar drug names can result in dispensing errors. Match each generic name with the appropriate brand name:

1.	Acetohexamide	a.	Flexeril®
2.	Acetazolamide	b.	Marezine®
3.	Allopurinol	c.	Dymelor®
4.	Chlorpromazine	d.	Narcan®
5.	Chlorpropamide	e.	Diamox®
6.	Cyclizine	f.	Compazine®
7.	Cyclobenzaprine	g.	Trexan®
8.	Methyldopa	h.	Mellaril®
9.	Naltrexone	i.	Diabinese®
10.	Naloxone	j.	Aldomet®
11.	Prochlorperazine	k.	Thorazine®
12.	Thioridazine	l.	Zyloprim®

E. Aseptic technique:

1. Is used exclusively for the compounding of injectable preparations
2. Prevents cross-contamination between two or more drugs
3. May include the injection of ethyl alcohol into powdered additives to sterilize the preparations
4. May prevent some allergic reactions in patients receiving injectable drugs
5. Answers 2 and 4 are correct

F. The use of laminar airflow hoods:

1. Is required for the preparation of all injectable drugs
2. May be used in some pharmacies, depending on specific policies
3. Is not required for all pharmacies preparing injectable drugs
4. Eliminates the possibility of microbial contamination
5. Answers 2, 3, and 4 are correct

G. Chemotherapeutic agents used to treat neoplasms (cancer) must *always* be prepared:

1. Using aseptic technique
2. In a laminar airflow hood
3. Using caution in handling
4. In a vertical laminar airflow hood
5. All of the above answers are correct

Answers to sample questions appear on pages 109–110.

Section II

Maintaining Medication and Inventory Control Systems

Includes activities related to medication and supply purchasing, inventory control, and preparation and distribution of medications according to approved policies and procedures

Chapter Four

Medication Distribution and Inventory Control Systems

I. Key Terms and Concepts

A. Inventory

1. The pharmacy's products or merchandise (drugs, devices, etc.) that are available to meet future demand

B. Inventory control

1. A procedure whereby products are purchased in sufficient quantity to meet the anticipated demands of purchasers while controlling inventory size to generate optimal profits

C. Turnover rate

1. The number of times a product is purchased, sold, and replaced during a specific accounting period. Inventory turnover is also discussed in Chapter Eleven.

II. Ordering Pharmaceuticals, Durable Medical Equipment, Devices, and Supplies

A. Identifying products to be ordered

1. Determining which products to order is dependent upon the inventory purchasing procedures of each individual pharmacy. Factors that influence ordering decisions include expected inventory turnover rate, manufacturing sources of products, and the purchase price of a particular product.

B. Entering information on products to be ordered

1. Pharmaceuticals

a. Drug name and manufacturer

(1) Generic name/manufacturer name

(2) Trade name if applicable

b. Strength and dosage form of medication (tablets, capsules, solutions, suspensions, injections, suppositories, etc.)

c. Type of packaging (unit dose or bulk packaging)

d. Quantity contained in unit desired (e.g.,100's, 16 oz.)

e. Number of units

2. Equipment, devices, and supplies

a. Name and manufacturer of product

b. Strength or size (if applicable) of product

c. Quantity contained in unit desired

d. Number of units

e. Other information as required

C. Identifying appropriate sources. Appropriate sources for various products are determined by each pharmacy's ordering policies.

1. Wholesale drug distributors
2. Manufacturers
3. Other pharmacies

D. Expediting emergency orders

1. The technician should be knowledgeable about the timetables for delivery on goods ordered from various sources so that drugs needed quickly can be obtained from the most desirable source in accordance with pharmacy policies and procedures.
2. In an emergency, the usual preferred sources may not be feasible and the pharmacy may need to borrow the product from a nearby institution.

III. Receiving Goods

A. Verifying specifications on original purchase orders

1. Verifying products ordered vs. products received. To ensure that the correct product was sent by the manufacturer or wholesale distributor, the technician must carefully scrutinize the order and confirm that the

information is consistent in all the components: (a) the original purchase order or "want book," (b) the invoice received with the order, and (c) the products received in the order. The following information should be compared and verified in each of the components for appropriateness and accuracy:

a. Drug name and manufacturer
    (1) Generic name/trade name
b. Strength and dosage form of medication
c. Appropriateness of packaging type (e.g., unit-dose vs. bulk packaging)
d. Quantity contained in unit desired (e.g., 100's, 16 oz.)
e. Number of units received vs. ordered

2. Documenting receipt of goods
    a. Pharmaceuticals, durable medical equipment, devices, and supplies
        (1) Notations on the invoice indicating receipt of appropriate products, or shortages, are usually written by the technician.
    b. Controlled substances
        (1) Receipt of controlled substances may also be documented by the supervising pharmacist.

IV. Placing Pharmaceuticals, Durable Medical Equipment, Devices, and Supplies in Inventory

A. Products should be placed in inventory under proper storage conditions. The technician should be knowledgeable about which products require special storage conditions (e.g., refrigeration).

B. Products should be placed in inventory according to stock rotation procedures, with items that will expire soonest placed in front of items with later expiration dates.

V. Removing Pharmaceuticals, Durable Medical Equipment, Devices, and Supplies from Inventory

A. Identifying products to be removed from inventory

1. Expired and discontinued products
2. Slow-moving products
3. Recalled products

VI. Repackaging Medications in Anticipation of Prescriptions/ Medication Orders

A. Prepackaging finished dosage forms for dispensing (e.g., unit dose)

1. Most drugs may be obtained in unit-dose packaging, but technicians may be responsible for repackaging some products. The technician should be familiar with the pharmacy's policies and procedures for repackaging in order to prevent shortages.

VII. Compounding Medications in Anticipation of Prescriptions/ Medication Orders

A. Bulk compounding

1. Compounds not commercially available may be prescribed and dispensed on a regular basis. In order to avoid the time-consuming activity of compounding the medication for each order, a large quantity may be prepared in advance in anticipation of future prescription or medication orders. The technician should be familiar with the pharmacy's policies and procedures for bulk compounding in order to prevent shortages.

VIII. Maintaining Record-Keeping Systems for Changes Affecting Inventory Levels of Pharmaceuticals, Durable Medical Equipment, Devices, and Supplies

A. Recalls and returns

1. Documenting recalls and returns may require entering the following information into the inventory records:
   a. Date the product was removed from inventory
   b. Information to identify the product
      (1) Pharmaceuticals
         (a) Drug name, strength, dosage form, and quantity removed

(2) Equipment, devices, and supplies

(a) Product name, size, and any other pertinent information for identification.

c. Manufacturer of the product

d. Lot number or identification number

e. Purpose for removing the drug from inventory (e.g., manufacturer recall)

f. Initials of technician and supervising pharmacist

g. Other information as required by pharmacy policies

B. Repackaging and bulk compounding of pharmaceuticals

1. Documenting repackaging and bulk compounding may require entering the following information into the inventory records:

a. Date the drug was removed from bulk inventory into the repackaged form or compounded product

b. Drug name, strength, dosage form, and quantity used

c. Lot number

d. Initials of technician and supervising pharmacist

e. Other information as required by pharmacy policies

IX. Maintaining Records of Controlled Substances

A. Recording controlled substances received and stored

1. Documentation of this function may require the following information:

a. Date the drug was received

b. Drug name, strength, dosage form, and quantity received

c. Initials of technician and supervising pharmacist

d. Other information as required by pharmacy policies

B. Recording controlled substances removed from inventory

1. Documentation of this function may require the following information:

a. Date the drug was removed from inventory

b. Drug name, strength, dosage form, and quantity removed

c. Lot number

d. Purpose for removing the drug from inventory (e.g., manufacturer recall)

e. Initials of technician and supervising pharmacist

f. Other information as required by pharmacy policies

X. Maintaining Policies and Procedures to Deter Theft and/or Drug Diversion

A. Drug theft and drug diversion are synonymous terms for illegally obtaining any medication; however, the drugs usually affected are controlled substances. The term drug diversion is generally used to describe health professionals stealing narcotics for personal use.

B. Drugs are stolen for many reasons, but three reasons predominate:

1. Personal abuse or addiction
2. Another person's abuse or addiction
3. Resale

C. Pharmacy policies to deter theft often include the following:

1. Storing controlled substances in a locked cabinet
2. Conducting a physical inventory of controlled substances periodically and monitoring the inventory on an ongoing basis
3. Maintaining records on controlled substances (see IX, above)
4. Allowing only a licensed pharmacist into the pharmacy after hours for dispensing of medications

XI. Communicating Changes in Product Availability to Pharmacy Staff, Patients/Patients' Representatives, Physicians, and Other Health Care Professionals

A. Reasons for changes in product availability

1. Recalls
2. Formulary changes
3. Discontinued products
4. Manufacturer shortages

B. Methods for communicating product changes
   1. Personal communication
      a. Communicating with the patient or patient's representative
      b. Staff meetings
   2. Written communication
      a. Memorandum to staff and other health care professionals
      b. Pharmacy newsletter
      c. Institutional newsletter

XII. Collecting and Analyzing Data on the Quality of Pharmacy Products and Services

A. Routine monitoring of the pharmacy department's activities is necessary to ensure the quality of pharmacy products and services and serves to identify existing and potential problems. Quality assurance activities include the collection and analysis of data on product preparation and distribution processes including:
   1. Sterile product testing
      a. Evaluating processes used in the preparation and sterilization of products to ensure that sterile products are free from microbial contamination, particulate matter, and pyrogens. Various tests are used in this assessment.
   2. Packaging unit-dose medications
   3. Bulk compounding
   4. Drug distribution activities
      a. Evaluating accuracy in filling and checking unit-dose medication carts
   5. Record-keeping activities
      a. Evaluating or reviewing patient profiles, medication administration records, and other records related to the above processes

XIII. Chapter Summary

A. Monitoring medication distribution and inventory control systems is a primary responsibility of pharmacy technicians.

B. The technician should be knowledgeable about the pharmacy's policies and procedures related to ordering products, receiving goods, storing products in inventory, repackaging, bulk compounding, quality assurance activities, and record-keeping systems for all processes.

XIV. Questions for Discussion

A. What factors should be considered in determining which products should be ordered for the pharmacy?

B. What factors should be considered in determining what quantity of a particular product should be ordered?

C. What factors should be considered in identifying the appropriate supplier from which to order a particular product?

D. Discuss the differences between drug theft and drug diversion. What is the technician's role in deterring drug theft and diversion?

E. Describe specific methods for collecting and analyzing data on the quality of pharmacy products and services.

XV. Sample Questions

A. When medications are recalled by the manufacturer, all of the following steps should be followed except:

1. Remove the recalled product from inventory.
2. Destroy the remaining units of recalled product and document actions.
3. Notify patients who are using the medication.
4. Notify health care providers about the recall.
5. All of the above steps should be followed.

B. True or false?

1. In institutional practice, all medications that are not available in unit-dose packaging must be repackaged.
2. Schedule II controlled substances may not be repackaged into unit-dose form.
3. To maintain an efficient inventory control system, slow-moving products should be removed from inventory.

C. Which of the following drugs should be stored in the refrigerator prior to dispensing?

1. Reconstituted amoxicillin suspension
2. Haloperidol solution
3. Sulfamethoxazole/trimethoprim suspension
4. Meperidine hydrochloride injection
5. All of the above medications should be stored in the refrigerator

D. Match the drug with the condition under which it should be stored:

1. Aspirin suppositories
2. Calcitonin-salmon nasal spray
3. Acetaminophen suppositories
4. Chlordiazepoxide injection
5. Diazepam injection
6. Lorazepam injection
7. L-hyoscyamine sulfate drops
8. Succinyl choline powder
9. Neosporin gentinourinary irrigant
10. Oral polio virus vaccine

a. Room temperature
b. Frozen
c. Refrigeration

Answers to sample questions appear on page 110.

Section III

Participating in the Administration and Management of Pharmacy Practice

Includes activities related to the administrative processes for the pharmacy practice site, including operations, human resources, facilities and equipment, and information systems

Chapter Five

Operations

I. Coordinating Communications Throughout the Practice Site and/or Service Area

A. Intradepartmental/interdepartmental communications

1. Verbal communication

a. Phone calls

(1) Phone calls may be addressed directly, or routed to the appropriate recipient. Some examples include:

(a) Route to pharmacist when physician calling

(b) Route to pharmacist when R.N. is calling with a new prescription or medication order.

(c) Route to other appropriate recipient (e.g., other technicians, pharmacy directors, administrators, etc.), depending on the specific type of information (e.g., change in I.V. orders, patient discharge, etc.) to be communicated.

(d) Accept calls from physicians or their representatives to authorize refills.

b. Interpersonal communication

(1) Accepting, communicating, and transmitting messages and information to, and from, those involved.

2. Written communication

a. Route faxes to appropriate recipients

b. Process prescriptions and medication orders

c. Route other written communications

B. Participating in meetings

1. Obtaining feedback regarding the performance of the practice site and/or service area

II. Monitoring the Practice Site and/or Service Area for Compliance with Federal, State, and Local Laws, Regulations, and Professional Standards

III. Implementing and Monitoring Policies and Procedures for Environmental Safety

A. Sanitation management

B. Hazardous waste handling (e.g., needles)

C. Infection control (e.g., protective clothing)

IV. Performing and Recording Routine Sanitation, Maintenance, and Calibration of Equipment

A. Equipment must be cleaned, sanitized, maintained, and calibrated at regularly scheduled intervals (or more often as necessary) to prevent contamination and to ensure proper performance.

B. Policies and procedures established for the cleaning and maintenance of equipment must be followed.

C. Records should be kept of equipment cleaning, maintenance, and inspection.

V. Maintaining a Manual or Computer-Based Information System

A. Manual and computer-based information systems are used to perform job-related activities, including:

1. Processing prescriptions and medication orders
2. Inventory control
3. Controlled-substances tracking
4. Updating drug prices

5. Administrative functions
    a. Workload and productivity tracking
    c. Drug utilization review
    e. Third-party authorization, billing, and reconciliation

VI. Maintaining Software for Computerized Systems

A. Automated dispensing technology

B. Point-of-care drug dispensing cabinets

VII. Personnel Functions

A. Perform or contribute to employee evaluations

B. Establish, implement, and monitor policies and procedures

VIII. Chapter Summary

A. Technicians should be knowledgeable about the activities, policies, and procedures related to the administrative processes for the pharmacy practice site including how and when to perform routine maintenance and calibration of equipment, monitoring the practice site for compliance with regulations and professional standards, and maintaining the pharmacy's information systems.

IX. Questions for Discussion

A. Discuss methods for coordinating communications throughout the practice site and/or service area.

B. Describe the various functions that can be managed and tracked using computer-based information systems.

X. Sample Questions

A. The pharmacy technician's role includes monitoring all of the above except:

1. Compliance with federal, state, and local laws
2. Compliance with regulations related to the handling of controlled substances
3. Policies and procedures for environmental safety
4. Quality control procedures used in the pharmacy
5. All of the above are included in the technician's responsibilities

B. Which of the following instruments should be routinely calibrated?

1. Prescription balance
2. Laminar airflow hood
3. Graduated cylinder
4. Mortar and pestle
5. All of the above answers are correct

Answers to sample questions appear on page 110.

Section IV

Pharmaceutical Calculations

Includes mathematical calculations related to the pharmacy practice site, including calculation of doses and injection flow rates, conversions between units of measurement, percentage preparations, reducing and enlarging formulas, and determining charges for prescriptions and medication orders

Chapter Six

Fractions, Decimals, and Roman Numerals

I. Fractions

A. Components of fractions

1. Example: 5/8

Numerator	5
Fraction line	—
Denominator	8

B. Types of common fractions

1. Proper fractions
   a. Proper fractions are fractions with a smaller numerator than denominator.
      (1) Example: 5/8
2. Improper fractions
   a. Improper fractions are fractions with a larger numerator than denominator.
      (1) Example: 8/5
   b. Improper fractions should be reduced to a mixed number.
      (1) Example: 8/5 should be reduced to $1\frac{3}{5}$
3. Simple fractions
   a. Simple fractions are proper fractions reduced to lowest terms.
      (1) Example: 15/24 = 5/8

4. Complex fractions

 a. Complex fractions are "fractions of fractions," where both the numerator and denominator are fractions.

 (1) Example: $\dfrac{5/8}{1/2}$

C. Reducing fractions to lowest terms

1. In reducing fractions, the fraction maintains its value but changes its form. Reduction of a fraction to lowest terms is accomplished by dividing both the numerator and denominator by the largest multiple that is common to both terms.

 a. Example: 15/24 is reduced to 5/8 by dividing both numerator and denominator by 3:

$$\frac{15 \div 3}{24 \div 3} \begin{matrix} = 5 \\ = 8 \end{matrix}$$

D. Five rules for calculating with fractions

1. Understand the impact of multiplying or dividing the numerator and/or denominator by a whole number.

Example: 4/8

$$\frac{4 \times 2}{8} = \frac{8}{8} = 1 \qquad \frac{4}{8 \times 2} = \frac{4}{16} = \frac{1}{4}$$

$$\frac{4 \div 2}{8} = \frac{2}{8} = \frac{1}{4} \qquad \frac{4}{8 \div 2} = \frac{4}{4} = 1$$

2. Convert mixed numbers or whole numbers to improper fractions before performing calculations with other fractions.

 a. Example: $2\,{}^{7}\!/\!_{8}$ = 23/8

3. When adding or subtracting fractions, make sure all fractions have a common denominator (i.e., a number into which all denominators may be divided an even number of times).

 a. Example: 3/4, 5/8, 1/2 may be written as 6/8, 5/8, 4/8

4. Convert answers that are improper fractions back to whole numbers or mixed numbers.

 a. Example: 15/3 = 5

5. Convert answers to lowest terms

   a. Example: 16/32 = 8/16 = 4/8 = 2/4 = 1/2

E. Adding and subtracting fractions

1. All fractions must first be converted so that they have a common denominator. The numerators are then added or subtracted.

   a. Example: 1/2 + 5/6 + 3/8 = 12/24 + 20/24 + 9/24 = 41/24 = $1\frac{17}{24}$

   b. Example: 13/32 – 3/8 = 13/32 – 12/32 = 1/32

F. Multiplying fractions

1. Unlike addition and subtraction, multiplication of fractions does not require common denominators. Multiply numerators by numerators and denominators by denominators.

   a. Example: $9\frac{2}{7}$ × 3/4 = 65/7 × 3/4 = 195/28 = $6\frac{27}{28}$

G. Dividing fractions

1. Invert the divisor and multiply the fractions.

   a. Example: 11/12 ÷ 1/6 = 11/12 × 6/1 = 66/12 = $5\frac{1}{2}$

   b. Example: $10\frac{3}{5}$ ÷ $2\frac{1}{10}$ = 53/5 ÷ 21/10 = 53/5 × 10/21 = 530/105 = $5\frac{5}{105}$ = $5\frac{1}{21}$

II. Decimals

A. Converting decimals to fractions

1. Decimal fractions are fractions with denominators of 10 and/or multiples of 10.

   a. A decimal number with one digit to the right of the decimal point is expressed in "tenths."

      (1) Example: 0.7 = 7/10

   b. A decimal number with two digits to the right of the decimal point is expressed as "hundredths."

      (1) Example: 0.27 = 27/100

   c. Follow the same rule as more digits are added to the right of the decimal point.

      (1) Example: 0.0365 = 365/10,000

B. Converting fractions to decimals

1. To convert common fractions to decimal fractions, divide the numerator by the denominator.

   a. Example: 3/4 = 0.75

   b. Example: $1\frac{5}{8}$ = 13/8 = 1.625

C. Adding, subtracting, multiplying, and dividing decimals

1. When adding, subtracting, multiplying, and dividing decimals and common fractions, convert all terms to the same system before performing the calculation.

   a. Example: 25/100 + 1.005 = 0.25 + 1.005 = 1.255

III. Roman Numerals

A. Primary roman numeral units

SS = 1/2
I or i = 1
V = 5
X = 10
L = 50
C = 100
D = 500
M = 1000

B. Eight rules of roman numerals

1. When a numeral is repeated, its value is repeated.
   a. Example: XX = 10 + 10 = 20
2. A numeral may not be repeated more than three times.
   a. Example: XL = 40 not XXXX
3. V, L, and D are never repeated. VV is incorrect.
4. When a smaller numeral is placed before a larger numeral, it is subtracted from the larger numeral.
   a. Example: XC = 100 – 10 = 90
5. When a smaller numeral is placed after a larger numeral, it is added to the larger numeral.
   a. Example: CX = 100 + 10 = 110
6. V, L, and D are never subtracted. VX is incorrect.
7. Never subtract more than one numeral.
   a. Example: VIII = 8 not IIX

8. Use I before V and X (only the next two highest numerals). The same is true for X and C (X before L and C; C before D and M).

IV. Sample Questions

A. Reduce the following fractions to lowest terms:

1. 10/75 = _____
2 8/16 = _____
3. 3/15 = _____
4. 60/186 = _____

B. Convert the following numbers to improper fractions:

1. 5 = _____
2. $3\frac{2}{3}$ = _____

C. Convert the following groups of fractions into groups of fractions with common denominators:

1. 15/32, 3/16, 7/64 = _____, _____, _____
2. 3/4, 7/8, 5/12 = _____, _____, _____

D. Convert 15/4 into a whole or mixed number: 15/4 = _____

E. 3/4 + $1\frac{1}{8}$ = _____

F. $7\frac{5}{8} - 1\frac{1}{3}$ = _____

G. $1\frac{3}{4} \times 3$ = _____

H. 1/2 ÷ 5 = _____

I. 3/16 ÷ $1\frac{1}{2}$ = _____

J. Convert the following decimal numbers to fractions:

1. 0.07 = _____
2. 0.077 = _____
3. 5.0125 = _____

K. Convert the following fractions to decimal numbers:

1. 3/8 = _____
2. $2\frac{7}{13}$ = _____

L. Perform the following calculations:

1. $3.75 - 1/2 =$ _____
2. $3/4 \times 2.5 =$ _____
3. $2\frac{3}{8} \div 0.5 =$ _____

M. Express the following numbers as roman numerals:

1. 29 = _____
2. 47 = _____
3. 86 = _____
4. 1154 = _____

N. Express the following roman numerals as Arabic numerals:

1. LXXVIII = _____
2. CXIII = _____
3. XCIV = _____
4. MCMLXI = _____

O. How many 0.0125 grain doses can be made from 3/8 grains of a drug?

P. How many ounces of boric acid would be left in an 8-ounce bottle if you dispensed 2 prescriptions each containing $1\frac{1}{4}$ ounces of boric acid and 3 additional prescriptions each containing 1.75 ounces from the bottle?

Q. How many 1/40 grain tablets would provide 1/200 grain of a drug?

R. How many 1/400 grain nitroglycerin tablets would provide 1/150 grain of nitroglycerin?

S. If 10 patients each receive XLIV mg of a drug, how many total mg (in Roman numerals) would all the patients receive?

Answers appear on pages 110–111.

Chapter Seven

Calculating Percentage and Ratio Strength

I. Percentage

A. Percent and its corresponding sign (%) mean "parts in one hundred."

1. Example: 40% may be expressed as:

   a. 40 parts in a 100, or

   b. 40/100, or

   c. 0.40, or

   d. 2/5 (40/100 = 4/10 = 2/5)

B. Converting percents to decimals

1. To change percents to decimals, remove the percent sign and move the decimal two places to the left.

   a. Example: 58% = 58/100 or 0.58

      72% = 72/100 or 0.72

C. Converting decimals and fractions to percents

1. Converting a decimal to a percent

   a. To convert a decimal to a percent, move the decimal two places to the right and add the percent sign.

      (1) Example: 0.17 = 17%

D. Percent expressed as a ratio

1. A ratio is the relationship or comparison of two like quantities.

   a. Example: 1/2 expressed as a ratio would be 1:2 or "1 part in two parts." This can also be expressed as:

      (1) a decimal (0.5), or

      (2) a percent (50%)

2. Converting a fraction to a percent

   a. To convert a fraction to a percent, reduce the fraction to a decimal and then move the decimal two places to the right and add the percent sign.

      (1) Example: 1/2 = 0.50 = 50%

II. Ratio and Proportion

A. Proportion

1. A proportion is the expression of the equality of two ratios or fractions. Most pharmacy calculations can be done using the principles of ratio and proportion.

B. Basic algebraic expression

1. The simplest algebraic form for a ratio and proportion is:

$$A/B = C/D, \text{ or } A:B = C:D$$

C. Solving for an unknown

1. By setting two equal ratios together, you may easily solve for an unknown if you know three terms of a proportion.

   a. Example: 3/5 = x/15

   This can be restated as, "if there are 3 parts in 5 parts, then there are x parts in 15 parts."

   Cross multiply to get: 5(x) = 45

   Rearrange the equation to: (x) = 45/5

   Divide to get the solution: x = 45/5 = 9

   Therefore, 3/5 = 9/15, or "3 parts in 5 parts is equivalent to 9 parts in every 15 parts."

III. Sample Questions

A. Convert the following:

1. 72% = 72/100 = 0.______
2. 0.35 = 35% = ______/100 = 7/___
3. 25% = 25/100 = ______:100
4. 0.182 = ______%
5. 3/8 = 0.______ = ______%

B. Using the principles of ratio and proportion, solve the following:

1. If 10 lb. of drug cost $200, what would 2 pounds cost?
2. How many pounds could you buy for $25?
3. What would 10 oz. cost (16 oz. per 1 lb.)?

C. A formula for 1000 tablets contains 11.5 grams of an antihistamine. How many grams of the antihistamine should be used to prepare 475 tablets?

D. A cough syrup contains 5 mg of a drug in each 15 ml dose. How many milligrams of drug would be contained in a 480 ml bottle of syrup?

E. If 2 tablets contain 650 mg of acetaminophen, how many milligrams would be contained in a bottle of 100 tablets?

F. If 7 tablets contain 35 mg of diazepam, how many tablets would contain 1500 mg?

G. If a patient pays $0.58 per tablet for 90 tablets, how much does the entire prescription cost?

H. How many grams of codeine sulfate would be required to prepare 20 capsules, each containing 0.0325 grams of codeine sulfate?

I. How much would 100 lb. of a chemical cost if 385 pounds cost $795?

J. How many kg would a 173 lb. patient weigh if there are 2.2 lb. in every kg?

K. If a penicillin solution contains 6 million units of penicillin in 10 ml, how many units would be contained in a 0.5 ml dose?

L. If a patient receives 5 ml of intravenous fluid per minute, how much fluid would the patient receive each hour?

M. How many milligrams of amoxicillin would a patient receive in one week if the patient receives 750 mg each day?

N. If a syringe contains 28 mg of drug in 3 ml how many milligrams of the drug would a patient receive if 1.2 ml is administered?

O. If a 480 ml bottle of 10% potassium chloride solution contains 10 grams of potassium chloride in every 100 ml of solution, how much potassium chloride will a patient receive from a 15 ml dose of the solution?

P. In the above question, how much would the bottle of potassium chloride cost if the 15 ml dose cost $0.28?

Answers appear on page 111.

Chapter Eight

Pharmaceutical Systems of Measurement

I. Measurement of Length, Weight, and Volume

A. Three systems of measurement are used in pharmacy:

1. Metric system measures weight, volume, and length
2. Apothecary system measures weight and volume
3. Avoirdupois system measures weight only

II. Metric System

A. Primary units (subdivided by multiples of 10)

1. Length: meter (m)
2. Volume: liter (L or l)
3. Weight: gram (g)

B. Common prefixes

1. "Increasing" prefix
   a. "Kilo-" (1000) is the most common "increasing" prefix
      (1) Example: 1 kilogram (kg) = 1000 g
2. "Decreasing" prefixes
   a. "milli-" (1/1000)
      (1) Example: 1 milligram (mg) = 0.001 g (1/1000 g)
      (2) Example: 1 gram = 1000 mg
   b. "Micro-" (1/1,000,000)
      (1) Example: 1 microgram (mcg or µg) = 0.000001 g
      (2) Example: 1 gram = 1,000,000 mcg

III. Apothecary System

A. Weight

1. Scruples 1 scruple = 20 grains (gr.)
2. Drams 1 dram = 3 scruples
3. Ounces 1 ounce = 8 drams
4. Pounds 1 pound = 12 ounces

B. Volume

1. Fluid dram 1 fluid dram = 60 minims
2. Fluid ounce 1 fluid ounce = 8 fluid drams
3. Pint 1 pint (pt) = 16 fluid ounces
4. Quart 1 quart (qt) = 2 pints
5. Gallon 1 gallon = 4 quarts

IV. Avoirdupois System

A. Weight

1. Ounce (oz.) 1 ounce = 437.5 grains (gr.)
2. Pound (lb.) 1 pound = 16 oz.

V. Common Conversions Between Systems

A. "Rounded-off" conversion factors

1. Weight

   a. 1 gram (g) = 15.4 grains (gr.)

   b. 1 grain (gr.) = 65 milligrams (mg)

   c. 1 pound (lb.) = 454 grams (g)

   d. 1 kilogram (kg) = 2.2 pounds (lb.)

2. Volume

   a. 1 fluid ounce = 30 milliliters (ml)

   b. 1 pint = 16 fluid ounces = 480 ml (Note: Sometimes the label on a pint bottle will read 473 ml instead of 480 ml. This is because a fluid ounce actually contains 29.57 ml but is frequently rounded to 30 ml.)

   c. 1 gallon = 4 quarts = 8 pints = 128 fluid oz. = 3840 ml

VI. Temperature Conversions

A. Converting degrees centigrade to degrees Fahrenheit

1. °F = 32 + 9/5°C

a. Example: 25°C

32 + 9/5 (25) = 77°F

B. Converting degrees Fahrenheit to degrees centigrade

1. °C = 5/9 (°F – 32)

a. Example: 32°F

5/9 (32 – 32) = 0°C

VII. Sample Questions

A. Convert the following metric system units:

1. 225 kilometers = ________ m
2. 525 g = ________ kg
3. 5 g = ________ mg = ________ mcg
4. 350 ml = ________ liters

B. Calculate the following using the apothecary system:

1. 3 scruples = 1 dram = ______ gr.
2. 8 drams = 1 ounce = ______ scruples = ______ gr.
3. 12 oz. = 1 pound = _____ drams = _____ scruples = _____ gr.
4. 8 fluid drams = 1 fluid ounce = ______ minims
5. 16 fluid ounces = 1 pint = _____ fluid drams
6. 2 pints = 1 quart = _____ fluid ounces
7. 4 quarts = 1 gallon = _____ pints = _____ fluid ounces

C. In the avoirdupois system:

1. 16 ounces = 1 pound = ________ gr.

D. What unit of weight has the same value in both the apothecary and avoirdupois systems—grain, pound, or ounce?

E. What measurement of volume do the apothecary and avoirdupois systems have in common?

F. What units do the apothecary and avoirdupois systems have in common with the metric system?

G. Using the "rounded-off" conversion factor for weight, fill in the blanks:

1. 1 grain = ______ g = ______ mg
2. 1 oz. = ______ gr. = ______ g
3. 1 lb. = ______ oz. = ______ g = ______ gr. = ______ kg
4. 1 ounce (apothecary) = ______ gr. = ______ g
5. 1 kg = ______ lb.

H. Using the "rounded-off" conversion factor for volume, fill in the blanks:

1. 1 pint = ______ fluid ounces = ______ milliliters (ml)
2. 1 gallon = ______ fluid ounces = ______ ml = ______ liters

I. Convert 20°C to Fahrenheit.

J. Convert 212°F to centigrade.

K. How many 325 mg aspirin tablets can be prepared from ½ kg of aspirin?

L. How many kg would a 246 lb. patient weigh?

M. A 10 ml vial contains 40 mg of a drug. How many mcg would be administered by injection of 2 ml of the drug?

N. If a physician orders 10 g of drug per liter, how many gr. would be in 250 ml?

Answers appear on pages 112–113.

Chapter Nine

Dosage Calculations

I. Basic Principles in Dosing

A. Key terms and concepts

1. Dose

   a. The quantity of a drug taken by a patient is known as the dose. The dose may be expressed as a "daily" dose, "single" dose, or even a "total" dose, which refers to all of the drug taken throughout therapy. "Daily" doses may be given once daily, which is a "single" dose, or may be divided throughout the day.

2. Dosage regimen

   a. A dosage regimen refers to the schedule of medication administration (e.g., every four hours, three times a day, at bedtime).

B. Doses vary tremendously due to differences in drug potency; routes of administration; the patients age, weight, kidney and liver functions, etc. Many factors can enter into establishing a correct dose, and many dispensing errors are related to administering the wrong dose. Pharmacy technicians can contribute to patient care by being familiar with appropriate doses of medications and by being able to calculate doses to check questionable orders.

II. Manufacturer's Recommended Dose

A. Manufacturers of medications establish the normal doses of drugs through research. This information can be obtained from numerous sources including package inserts, *Physician's Desk Reference (PDR), USP DI, Facts and Comparisons*, and others. These doses are usually listed as milligrams or milliliters per kilogram (or lb.) of body weight. The calculation of doses can usually be performed by simply using the principles of ratio and proportion.

1. Example: The dose of a drug is 10 mg per kg of body weight. How much would you give a 220 lb. man?
    a. Step 1: 2.2 lb./1 kg = 220 lb./x

       x = 100 kg of body weight

    b. Step 2: 10 mg drug/1 kg = x/100 kg

       x = 1000 mg = 1 g of drug

III. Household Equivalents

A. Household equivalents are measurements frequently used in dosing. They are referred to as "household equivalents" because they are measures frequently found in homes (teaspoons, pints, tablespoons, etc.).

1. 1 teaspoonful (tsp.) = 5 ml
2. 1 tablespoonful (tbsp.) = 15 ml
3. 1 fluid ounce = 30 ml

IV. Flow Rate Calculations

A. Flow rate calculations are normally used for intravenous solutions and can be done by "multiple" ratio and proportion calculations.

1. Example: If an I.V. order is for 500 ml of D_5 NS to be given over 4 hours (240 minutes), and the I.V. set delivers 15 drops per ml, what would be the flow rate?

Step 1: $\frac{15\ \text{gtt}}{1\ \text{ml}} = \frac{x}{500\ \text{ml}}$ x = 7500 total drops (gtts)

Step 2: $\frac{7500\ \text{gtt}}{240\ \text{min}} = \frac{x}{1\ \text{min}}$ x = 31 gtts/min

NOTE: Another method for calculating flow rates is by using the following formula:

$$\frac{(\text{ml/hr})\ (\text{gtts/ml})}{60\ \text{min/hr}} = \text{flow rate in gtts/min}$$

Using the above example:

$$\frac{(500\ \text{ml}/4\ \text{hrs})\ (15\ \text{gtts/ml})}{60\ \text{min/hr}} = 31\ \text{gtts/min}$$

V. Sample Questions

A. Solve the following using the principles of ratio and proportion:

1. 1 tbsp. = 15 ml = _____ tsp.
2. 1 fluid oz. = 30 ml = _____ tsp. = _____ tbsp.
3. 1 pt. = _____ fluid oz. = _____ ml = _____ tbsp. = _____ tsp.

B. A child's amoxicillin dose is 20 mg/kg/day in divided doses every 8 hours.

1. This could also be written as 20 mg/________lb./day.
2. How many grams of amoxicillin would a 44-lb. child receive daily?
3. How many milligrams per dose?
4. Amoxicillin is available as an oral suspension (125 mg/5 ml). How many teaspoonsful should this child receive per dose?
5. How many teaspoonsful should this child receive per day?
6. How many milliliters would you dispense for 10 days of therapy?
7. How many fluid ounces would you dispense for 10 days of therapy?
8. How many doses would the patient receive in 7 days?

C. How many milliliters of a liquid laxative should be dispensed if the dose prescribed is for 1 tablespoonful qid for 3 days?

D. Flow rate calculations

1. If the flow rate for normal saline (NS) is 30 drops per minute over 6 hours, how many milliliters of NS would the patient receive (assuming 18 gtts/ml)?
2. How many grams of NaCl would be administered (NS = 0.9 g of NaCl per 100 ml)?

E. A drug is administered by infusion at the rate of 1 mcg/lb./minute for anesthesia. If a 90 kg man is to receive a total of 0.85 mg of the drug:

1. How long should the drug be infused?
2. If the drug is available in a strength of 2 mg/5 ml, how many milliliters would the patient receive per minute?
3. How many total milliliters would the patient receive?

F. How many milliliters of an injection containing 90 mg/ml of a drug should be administered to a 50 lb. child if the recommended dose is 6 mg per pound of body weight?

G. How many 125 mg antifungal tablets should be dispensed for a 100-lb. patient to provide a 30 day supply if the normal daily dose is 5 mg per pound of body weight?

H. An injectable antibiotic has a dose of 10 mg per kg of body weight. How many milliliters of a 125 mg/ml injection should be administered to a child weighing 66 lb.?

I. How many ml of digoxin injection 0.5 mg/2 ml would provide a 100 mcg dose?

J. A solution of sodium fluoride contains 1.1 mg/ml and has a dose of 15 drops. How many milligrams of sodium fluoride are in each dose if the dispensing dropper calibrates at 28 gtts/ml ?

Answers appear on pages 113–114.

Chapter Ten

Concentrations

I. Reducing and Enlarging Formulas

A. Pharmacists and technicians often have to prepare larger and/or smaller quantities than a recipe might call for.

1. Example: Recipe on a box for eight medium-size pancakes

Pancake mix	1 cup
Water	1/2 cup
Milk	1/4 cup
Eggs	2
Vegetable oil	2 tsp

a. How much milk would be needed to make 16 pancakes?

b. How many eggs are needed to make four pancakes?

The above problems can be solved by creating a factor using the amount the recipe calls for as a denominator and the amount desired as the numerator. Multiply this factor times each component in the recipe to "reduce" or "enlarge" the formula. In the above examples, the calculation would be:

$$\frac{16\text{ pancakes}}{8\text{ pancakes}} = 2\,(1/4\text{ cup of milk}) = 1/2\text{ cup of milk}$$

$$\frac{4\text{ pancakes}}{8\text{ pancakes}} = 1/2\,(2\text{ eggs}) = 1\text{ egg}$$

The problems can also be solved using the principles of ratio and proportion:

$$\frac{1/4\text{ cup of milk}}{8\text{ pancakes}} = \frac{x}{16\text{ pancakes}} \qquad x = 1/2\text{ cup}$$

$$\frac{2\text{ eggs}}{8\text{ pancakes}} = \frac{x}{4\text{ pancakes}} \qquad x = 1\text{ egg}$$

II. Concentrations and Dilutions

A. Concentration may be expressed as a percentage. There are three types of percentages:

1. Weight-in-weight (w/w) percentage preparations

   a. Weight-in-weight percentage is used when the final product is a solid (powder, ointment, etc.), and the component you are measuring the percentage of is also a solid. Units in the numerator and denominator must be the same (lb./lb., gr./gr., etc.).

      (1) Example: 2 g of sulfur in 100 g of a final ointment would be 2 g/100 g = 0.02 = 2% w/w

2. Volume-in-volume (v/v) percentage preparations

   a. Volume-in-volume percentage is used when the final product is a liquid (solution) and the component you are measuring the percentage of is also a liquid. Units in the numerator must be the same as in the denominator (ml/ml, pt/pt, etc.).

      (1) Example: 5 ml of a flavoring oil in 100 ml of mouthwash would be 5 ml/100 ml = 0.05 = 5% v/v

3. Weight-in-volume (w/v) percentage preparations

   a. Weight-in-volume percentage is used when the final product is a liquid as indicated by the (v) in the denominator (e.g., suspensions) and the component you are measuring the percentage of is a solid as indicated by the (w) in the numerator. The numerator is always in grams and the denominator is always in milliliters (this differs from w/w and v/v percents, where the units could vary but have to be the same in both the numerator and denominator).

      (1) Example: 17 g of drug K in 100 ml of a final solution would be 17 g/100 ml = 0.17 or 17% w/v

B. Ratio strength preparations

1. Ratios are just another way of expressing a percent (remember that percent means parts per 100). A 5% w/w product is 5 parts per 100 parts or 5:100. A 20% v/v solution is 20 parts per 100 parts or 20:100 (this could mean 20 ml of drug in 100 ml of solution or 20 L in

100 L, etc.). A 15% w/v solution means 15 g of drug in 100 ml of solution or 15:100. Ratio strength calculations are performed like percentage calculations.

a. Example: 5% w/v = 5 g in 100 ml = 1 g in 20 ml = 1:20

2. Ratios should always be reduced so that the number "1" is written to the left of the colon (e.g., 1:100, not 2:200, even though these ratios are equal).

a. Example: 3:15 could also be written:

$$\frac{3}{15} = \frac{1}{x}$$

$$x = 5 \text{ so } 3:15 = 1:5$$

C. Stock solutions

1. Stock solutions are concentrated solutions from which weaker strength solutions can be easily made.

D. Dilutions of stock preparations

1. A dilution is performed when you take a certain percentage solution and add a 0% diluent to decrease the percentage concentration.

a. Example: How much water would you add to 100 ml of a 15% potassium chloride solution to get a 5% final product?
This problem cannot be solved by simple ratio and proportion because you are looking for an inverse relationship (i.e., the more solvent we add, the *lower* the percentage).

(1) Easy method:

$$(\text{old volume})(\text{old }\%) = (\text{new volume})(\text{new percent})$$

$$(100 \text{ ml})(15\%) = (x)(5\%)$$

$$\frac{(100 \text{ ml})(15\%)}{(5\%)} = x$$

$$x = 300 \text{ ml}$$

Note: 300 ml is the final and total dilution you have made by adding 100 ml of 15% KCl to a certain volume of water. It is not the amount of water added.

Answer: 300 ml final solution – 100 ml of 15% = 200 ml of H_2O added.

III. Alligations

A. Alligation alternate

1. Basic principles

   a. This technique is used for making dilutions when the diluent is zero percent or higher. Previous dilution examples used a zero percent diluent only.

   b. You can only dilute to an intermediate percent (i.e., you cannot add 10% to 20% and get a percent higher than 20% or lower than 10%). The final product will be somewhere between 10% and 20%.

2. Examples

   a. If you need a 10% sulfur ointment and only have 5% and 20% ointments available, use the alligation alternate method to determine how many "parts" of each will be needed to get the 10% final product. "Parts" can have any value (ml, gr., pinches, etc.) and all the "parts," when added together, will equal the total "parts" of the final product, in this case the 10% ointment.

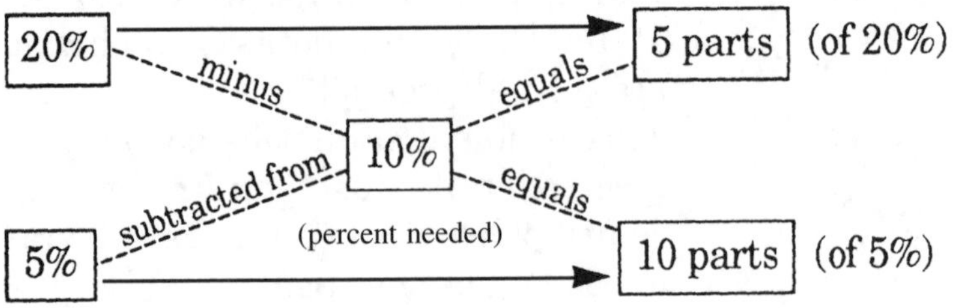

   Subtract 5% from 10% to get 5 parts. Subtract 10% from 20% to get 10 parts.

   So the ratio is 5 parts of 20%:10 parts of 5%.

   b. From the previous example prepare 1 kg of the 10% sulfur ointment.

   Step 1: Add the parts, i.e., 5 + 10 = 15 parts (Note: the 15 parts represents the total quantities of the 20% and 5% ointments that are being combined. The "new" product which is a 10% ointment is equal to 15 parts.)

   Step 2: 15 parts/1000 g = 10 parts/x x = 667 g (of 5% ointment)

Step 3: 15 parts/1000 g = 5 parts/x   x = 333 g (of 20% ointment)

Note: Step 3 can be skipped by simply subtracting 667 from 1000

Note: To compound 1000 g of 10%, add 667 g of 5% ointment to 333 g of 20% ointment.

B. Alligation medial

1. This method is used to obtain the average strength of a mixture of two or more substances whose concentration and percent strength are already known. This can also be used to check an alligation alternate problem.

a. Example from the mixture in A.2. above:

Step 1:

$$\begin{array}{lcl} 5 \text{ parts} \times 20\% & = & 100 \text{ parts } \% \\ 10 \text{ parts} \times 5\% & = & 50 \text{ parts } \% \\ \hline 15 \text{ parts} & & 150 \text{ parts } \% \end{array}$$

Step 2:

$$\frac{150 \text{ parts } \%}{15 \text{ parts } \%} = 10\%$$

IV. Milliequivalents

A. Key terms and concepts

1. Electrolytes

a. Electrolytes are important for many bodily functions that require electrical activity such as nerve conduction and muscle contraction. Electrolyte replacement is usually ordered in units of milligrams or milliequivalents.

2. Milliequivalents

a. A milliequivalent (mEq) is equal to the millimoles of H^+ or OH^- that will react with 1 mmol of an ion or compound. When an atom has the valence of "one," a milliequivalent (mEq) is simply equal to the atomic weight of the atom (e.g., Na^+ = 23 so there are 23 mg/mEq). A molecule like sodium chloride (NaCl) has a molecular weight (MW) of 58.5. Therefore, 1 mEq = 58.5 mg, and when it dissociates, yields 1 mEq Na^+ and 1 mEq Cl^-.

B. Converting to milliequivalents

1. Example: If a solution contains 10 g of potassium chloride (KCl), how many mEq of K^+ does it contain? The atomic weight (AW) of K^+ = 39 and AW of Cl^- = 35.5. Therefore, the MW of KCl = 74.5

   74.5 mg = 1 mEq

   10 g = 10,000 mg

   74.5 mg/1 mEq = 10,000 mg/x = 134 mEq

C. Divalent and trivalent ions

1. Sometimes you will have an exception to the rule when you have divalent ions (e.g., Mg^{++}, Ca^{++}) and trivalent ions (e.g., Al^{+++}). In most cases when magnesium or calcium are involved in the molecule, 1 mEq is equal to 1/2 the molecular weight. With aluminum-containing products, 1 mEq is equal to 1/3 the molecular weight.

   a. Example: Calcium Chloride ($CaCl_2$)

   AW of Ca^{++} = 40 AW of Cl^- = 35.5
   40 + 35.5 + 35.5 = 111 mg total weight
   1 mEq = 111/2 (i.e., valence) = 55.5 mg

V. Dry Powders for Reconstitution

A. Many unstable medications are packaged as dry powders and must be dissolved in a solvent prior to dispensing. The most frequently encountered drugs requiring reconstitution are the antibiotics. In most cases, reconstitutions can be accomplished in three steps:

Step 1. Establish how much drug is in the vial or bottle.

Step 2. Calculate the powder volume displacement.

Step 3. Solve the problem using ratio and proportion.

a. Example 1: The label on a vial reads, "Add 9.2 ml of diluent to the vial to get 10 ml of a 100 mg/ml solution for injection." How many milliliters of the reconstituted solution would provide a 250 mg dose?

(1) Step 1: $\frac{100\text{ mg}}{1\text{ ml}} = \frac{x}{10\text{ ml}}$
x = 1000 mg/vial
(2) Step 2: not required at this point
(3) Step 3: $\frac{1000\text{ mg}}{10\text{ ml}} = \frac{250\text{ mg}}{x}$
x = 2.5 ml

Note: This can also be solved using the per milliliter concentration of 100 mg/1 ml: $\frac{100\text{ ml}}{1\text{ ml}} = \frac{250\text{ mg}}{x}$

b. How much of the diluted solution for injection in Example 1 would you measure to get the 250 mg dose if you accidentally reconstituted with 11 ml of diluent?

(1) Step 1: 1000 mg per vial

(2) Step 2: If 9.2 ml of diluent when mixed with the powder yields 10 ml, then the powder volume displacement is 0.8 ml, i.e., 10 – 9.2 = 0.8.

(3) Step 3: 0.8 ml of powder + 11 ml of diluent = 11.8 ml

$$\frac{1000\text{ mg} = 250\text{ mg}}{11.8\text{ ml} \quad x}$$
x = 2.95 ml

c. Example 2: You have been directed to reconstitute a 5 million unit vial of Drug A to a concentration of 500,000 units/ml. The drug has a powder volume displacement of 0.002 L. How many milliliters of diluent will you need to add to this vial?

(1) Step 1: 5,000,000 units per vial

(2) Step 2: 2 ml (given as 0.002 L)

(3) Step 3: If you want 500,000 units per 1 ml, then

$$\frac{500{,}000\text{ units}}{1\text{ ml}} = \frac{5{,}000{,}000\text{ units}}{x}$$

x = 10 ml (this is the total volume of the vial)
10 ml total volume – 2 ml powder volume displacement = 8 ml of diluent to be added

VI. Sample Questions

A. Answer questions 1–3 using the following recipe for benzyl benzoate lotion:

Benzyl benzoate	250 ml
Triethanolamine	5 g
Oleic acid	20 g
Purified water to make	1000 ml

1. How many grams of triethanolamine are required to make one gallon of benzyl benzoate lotion? How many milligrams?
2. How many grains of oleic acid are required to make one pint of benzyl benzoate lotion?
3. How many teaspoonsful of benzyl benzoate are there in 100 ml of the lotion?

B. What percentage of sulfur would be in a product that contains 2 g of sulfur in 120 grams of ointment?

1. How many milligrams of sulfur would be contained in 1 g of ointment?

C. What percentage of sulfur would be in a product containing 20 g of sulfur in 1 lb. of ointment?

D. What percentage sulfur ointment would result from *adding* 50 g of sulfur to 120 g of petrolatum?

1. What is the percentage of petrolatum in the ointment?

E. Ninety grams of 25% zinc oxide ointment would contain how many grams of zinc oxide?

F. What percentage of flavoring oil would be in a mouthwash that has two tablespoonsful of oil in one pint of mouthwash?

1. How many milliliters of oil would be in 60 ml of the mouthwash?

G. Calculate the percentage of a preparation containing 7 g of drug K in 5 fluid ounces of a final product.

H. Calculate the percentage of a preparation containing 1 lb. of drug K in one gallon of final product.

1. What is the ratio strength of the final product?

I. One pint of a 10% w/v suspension would contain ______ grams of drug.

1. One teaspoonful of this suspension would be what percent w/v?

J. One quart of a 1:50 w/v solution would be ______% and contain ______ g of active ingredient.

K. How many mg/ml would be in a 6% w/v solution?

1. What is the ratio strength of this solution?

L. A solution containing 2000 mg of a drug in 8 fluid ounces would be a _____% w/v solution or a _____ ratio strength solution and contain _____ mg/ml.

M. Convert 6:720 into a correctly written ratio strength.

1. Express this as a percentage strength.

N. What is the resulting percentage of benzalkonium chloride obtained from diluting one fluid ounce of 17% benzalkonium chloride to one pint?

1. What is the final ratio strength?
2. How many mg/ml are in the final dilution?
3. How many grams per teaspoonful are in the initial 17% solution?
4. What is the percentage strength of 1 teaspoonful of the 17% solution *added* to one tablespoonful of water?
5. How many grains of benzalkonium chloride are in one fluid ounce of 17% benzalkonium chloride?
6. How many grains of benzalkonium chloride are in the final one pint dilution?
7. If 100 ml of 1:200 drug solution is diluted to 1 L, what is the final ratio strength?
8. How many milligrams per teaspoonful doses are in the final dilution in question N.7?

O. Can you mix a 20% ointment with a 5% ointment to make a 10% ointment?

1. If yes, how many grams of each component would be required to make 1 lb. of a 10% ointment?
2. If yes, how many grams of 10% ointment could be made if you had only 30 g of 20% and plenty of 5%?

P. Can you mix a 20% ointment with a 15% ointment to make a 10% ointment?

1. If yes, how many grams of each component would be required to make 1 lb. of a 10% ointment?
2. If yes, how many grams of 10% ointment could be made if you had only 1 oz. of 20% and plenty of 15%?

Q. A liter of NS (0.9% sodium chloride) would contain ______ grams of sodium chloride and ______ mEq of sodium? (AW of Na^+ = 23; AW of Cl^- = 35.5)

R. If 100 ml of a solution contains 10 mEq of KCl, what is the percentage strength of potassium chloride? (MW of KCl = 74.5)

1. How many milligrams of KCl are required to prepare 1 L of the above solution?

S. How many milliequivalents of calcium are in a tablespoonful of a solution containing 250 mg of calcium chloride ($CaCl_2$)? (AW of Ca^{++} = 40; Cl^- = 35.5)

T. What is the percentage strength of calcium chloride in the above solution?

U. How many milliequivalents of aluminum are in 1 g of aluminum hydroxide Al $(OH)_3$? (AW of Al = 27; O = 16; H = 1)

V. Answer questions V. 1–3 using the following prescription for ampicillin suspension:

Rx Ampicillin 250 mg/5 ml Sig: 1 tsp qid × 10 d

1. How many milliliters would you dispense?
2. Assume that the instructions on the bottle of dry ampicillin powder for reconstitution require the addition of 160 ml of water to obtain the volume needed to correctly fill the prescription. What volume will the drug powder account for?
3. How many grams of ampicillin will the patient receive in one week?

W. The prescription below is a formula for one capsule to be extemporaneously compounded. How many 30 mg codeine sulfate tablets would be required to make 50 of these capsules?

Rx	
Acetylsalicylic acid	325 mg
Codeine sulfate	5 mg
Sig: 1 capsule q 4 h prn pain	

X. How many 250 mg erythromycin tablets would be required to compound the prescription below?

Rx	
E-Mycin	2%
Alcohol qs	150 ml

1. What is the ratio strength of 1 teaspoonful of the prescription?
2. How many milligrams are in each milliliter of the prescription?

Y. The instructions on a vial for reconstitution state, “Add 12.8 ml of diluent to make 15 ml of a 500 mg/ml solution.” You have on hand only 10 ml of the diluent, which you use for reconstitution.

1. How much drug is in the vial?
2. Does the total amount of drug in the vial change according to the amount of diluent added?
3. Does the amount of drug per milliliter vary with the amount of diluent added?
4. What is the powder volume displacement of the drug?
5. How many milliliters of the reconstituted solution, according to instructions on the vial, would provide a 2 g dose of the drug?
6. How many milliliters of the reconstituted solution made with 10 ml of diluent would provide a 2 g dose of the drug?

Z. What is the percent strength of coal tar in a mixture of 1/2 kg of 3% coal tar ointment and 1500 g of 10% coal tar ointment?

1. What is the ratio strength of the coal tar mixture?
2. How many grams of coal tar are in 1 lb. of this mixture?
3. Can a 1:50 coal tar ointment be prepared by mixing the 3% and 10% coal tar ointments?
4. How many grams of coal tar should be added to the coal tar mixture to obtain an ointment containing 18% coal tar?

Answers appear on pages 114–116.

Chapter Eleven

Commercial Calculations

I. Determining Charges for Prescriptions and Medication Orders

A. Cost

1. Cost is the total paid for an item or items received as noted on an invoice.

   a. Example: The invoice states that you purchased 1/2 dozen mugs at $1.50 each, for a total of $9.00.

   $$6 \times \$1.50 \text{ each} = \$9 \text{ or } \frac{1 \text{ mug}}{\$1.50} = \frac{6 \text{ mugs}}{x}$$

B. Selling price

1. The selling price is 100% of the amount you will receive for the sale of an item (this includes your cost plus whatever amount you want as a profit).

C. Markup

1. Markup may be defined as the difference between your cost for a product and its actual selling price.

   Selling price = Cost + Markup

2. Example: For 30 tablets costing $0.40 each for which you want to receive $0.10 profit per tablet:

   $$\text{Selling price} = (30 \times \$0.40) + (30 \times \$0.10) = \$15.00$$

   $$\text{or} \quad \$12.00 + \$3.00 = \$15.00$$

D. Percent markup

1. The percent markup must be qualified before it can be defined. It must be stated as "percent markup on the selling price" or as "percent markup on the cost" in order to determine its true meaning. In retail practice, "percent markup" usually means percent of sales and not of cost.

a. From the previous example, percent markup based on cost would be:

$$\frac{\text{markup}}{\text{cost}} = \frac{\$3.00}{\$12.00} = 0.25 = 25\%$$

E. Percent gross profit

1. This is the percent based on the selling price instead of the cost.

a. Example:

$$\text{Percent gross profit} = \frac{\text{markup}}{\text{selling price}} = \frac{\$3.00}{\$15.00} = 0.20 = 20\%$$

F. Overhead

1. It is important to consider overhead to determine the true profit of a business. Overhead includes operating costs such as utilities, taxes, insurance, and technician salaries.

G. Net profit

1. Net profit can be defined as:

a. Selling price – (cost of goods + overhead)

H. Inventory

1. The inventory includes all items on hand and their cost.

I. Turnover

1. Turnover refers to the number of times that merchandise is sold in a given length of time, normally one year.

II. Sample Questions

A. If you paid $.20 per capsule for a bottle containing 100 capsules, what was the total cost of the bottle of capsules?

1. If you wanted to make a $0.05 profit per capsule, what would be the selling price of one capsule?
2. What would be the selling price of 30 capsules?

B. If a drug costs $50 and the selling price is $60:

1. What is the markup?
2. What is the percent markup based on cost?
3. What is the percent gross profit?

Answers appear on pages 116–117.

Chapter 12

Practice Questions

1. Which of the following products is not commercially available?

   a. Allopurinol 100 mg tablets
   b. Prednisone 5 mg tablets
   c. Alprazolam 5 mg tablets
   d. Indinavir sulfate 200 mg capsules

2. How many milligrams of zephirin chloride are needed to prepare 3 L of 1:30,000 solution?

   a. 0.1
   b. 1
   c. 10
   d. 100

3. How many grams of bacitracin (500 units/g) should be used to prepare 1 kilogram of bacitracin ointment containing 250 units of bacitracin per gram?

   a. 100
   b. 500
   c. 1000
   d. 250,000

4. Patient profiles should be created for:

   a. Patients who have chronic diseases (e.g., diabetes, hypertension, etc.)
   b. Patients who have prescriptions filled at the pharmacy regularly
   c. Every patient who presents a prescription to the pharmacy
   d. Any patient who has had 3 or more prescriptions filled at the pharmacy within a 6-month period

5. How many milliliters of a drug would be needed to provide a 10,000 mcg dose from a vial containing 0.1 g/10 ml?

   a. 1
   b. 10
   c. 100
   d. 1000

6. How many milligrams of ephedrine sulfate should be used to prepare the following prescription?

Rx Sol. Ephedrine Sulfate ¼% 30 ml
Sig. Use as Directed

a. 0.075
b. 0.75
c. 7.5
d. 75

7. What is the generic name for Keftab?

a. Cefadroxil
b. Cefixime
c. Cephalexin
d. Ceftazadime

8. An order is received to administer 5 mEq of potassium acetate per hour. The bag of I.V. fluid contains 30 mEq per liter. How many drops per minute would be needed to provide the prescribed dose using a set that delivers 15 gtts/ml?

a. 3
b. 12
c. 42
d. 167

9. How many liters of a 0.9% aqueous sodium chloride solution can be made from 60 g of NaCl?

a. 6.67
b. 66.7
c. 667
d. 6,667

10. How many grams of a 5% sulfur ointment must be mixed with 180 g of 20% sulfur ointment to prepare an 8% sulfur ointment?

a. 45
b. 90
c. 180
d. 720

11. If 5 ml of diluent are added to a vial containing 2 g of a drug for injection resulting in a final volume of 5.8 ml, what is the concentration in mg/ml of the drug in the reconstituted solution?

a. 0.3
b. 345
c. 400
d. 2035

12. Which prescription instructions would require 17 tablets to be dispensed?

    a. One tab p.o. bid × 7 d
    b. One tab a.c. & h.s. × 4 d
    c. One tab t.i.d. × 3 d; one b.i.d. × 3 d; one q.d. × 3 d
    d. Two tabs b.i.d. × 2 d; two tabs q.d. × 3 d; one tab q.d. × 3 d

13. Which of the following is not considered a dosage form?

    a. Powder
    b. Inhalation
    c. Paste
    d. Lotion

14. How many milliliters per hour would be required to infuse a dopamine dose of 5 mcg/kg/min to a patient weighing 220 lb. if the dopamine is provided by a bag containing 800 mg/500 ml?

    a. 18.75
    b. 30.35
    c. 100.45
    d. 528.34

15. A physician prescribes 10 mg of a drug per kilogram of body weight once daily for 21 days for a patient weighing 264 lb. How many 200-mg tablets of the drug are required daily?

    a. 2
    b. 4
    c. 6
    d. 12

16. How many grams of potassium permanganate are required to prepare 2 quarts of 1:750 solution of potassium permanganate?

    a. 0.05
    b. 0.13
    c. 1.28
    d. 13

17. When the physician's instructions indicate that a drug should be taken sublingually, what directions might be included on the prescription label?

    a. Change the patch every 12 hours
    b. Chew the medication thoroughly
    c. Place the medication under the tongue until it dissolves
    d. Use 0.5 ml in 2 ml of normal saline every 4 hours as needed

18. The formula for zinc gelatin is:

Glycerin	400 g
Gelatin	150 g
Zinc Oxide	100 g
Purified Water	350 g

How much glycerin would be required to prepare 1 lb. of zinc gelatin?

a. 182 g
b. 192 g
c. 519 g
d. 1000 g

19. Which drug is used to treat patients with diabetes?

a. Micronase
b. Glycotrol
c. Glucophase
d. DiaBeta-trol

20. How many 1/2 pint bottles can be filled from a 2 gallon container of 10% potassium chloride?

a. 16
b. 32
c. 64
d. 128

21. A complete patient profile should include all of the following except:

a. Nonprescription medications the patient is currently using
b. Patient's annual income for reimbursement/payment information
c. The brand name or manufacturer of the drug dispensed to fill the prescription
d. Physical limitations and sociological factors specific to the patient

22. What is the percent alcohol contained in a mixture of 90 ml of elixir phenobarbital (14% alcohol), 100 ml of water, and 40 ml of high alcoholic elixir (78% alcohol)?

a. 8%
b. 19%
c. 26%
d. 64%

23. The technician must notify the pharmacist before modifying the patient profile in all cases except:

    a. The patient has experienced a stroke and has been prescribed a different antihypertensive medication
    b. The strength or dosage of insulin differs from the patient's previous prescription
    c. The patient is now covered by a new medical/prescription insurance company
    d. The patient has become pregnant since the last prescription was filled

24. If the dose of a drug is 35 mg/kg/day in six divided doses, how much would be given in each dose to a 38 lb. child?

    a. 17.3 mg
    b. 60.4 mg
    c. 101 mg
    d. 604 mg

25. How many micrograms of digoxin would be contained in 0.75 ml of an ampule labeled 0.5 mg/2 ml?

    a. 0.188
    b. 3.6
    c. 13.2
    d. 187.5

26. Patient information to be entered into the patient profile must include all of the following except:

    a. The pharmacist's signature confirming each item of information listed
    b. Blood pressure measurements taken by the technician
    c. Patient allergies
    d. Reimbursement mechanisms

27. How many grams of potassium chloride are used in making 1 L of a solution containing 3 mEq of potassium per teaspoonful? (MW of KCl = 74.5)

    a. 44.7
    b. 74.5
    c. 223.5
    d. 44,700

28. How many milliliters of 20% merthiolate solution should be diluted with water to make 600 ml of a 0.5% merthiolate solution?

a. 15
b. 178
c. 580
d. 24,000

29. Using proper aseptic technique requires that all intravenous solutions must be:

a. Filtered prior to dispensing
b. Prepared in a laminar flow hood
c. Administered in at least 50 ml of normal saline
d. Refrigerated immediately after compounding

30. How many grams of yellow mercuric oxide must be *added* to 30 g of 1% yellow mercuric oxide ointment to prepare a 5% ointment?

a. 0.8
b. 1.26
c. 28.9
d. 713

31. An elixir is to contain 500 μg of an alkaloid in each tablespoonful dose. How many milligrams of alkaloid would be required to prepare a liter of the elixir?

a. 3.33
b. 7.5
c. 33.3
d. 33,333

32. A prescription calls for 500 mg of tetracaine hydrochloride. If tetracaine hydrochloride costs $24.50 per 3 g, what is the cost of the quantity necessary to prepare the prescription?

a. $1.25
b. $2.85
c. $4.08
d. $147.72

33. How many milliliters of ampicillin 250 mg/5 ml should be dispensed to fill a prescription for 500 mg qid times 10 days?

a. 100
b. 150
c. 200
d. 400

34. An example of injectable drug cross-contamination that could cause a potentially fatal reaction would be:

a. Cefamandole-cefazolin
b. Gentamicin-amikacin
c. Ampicillin-Aminophylline
d. Meperidine-codeine

35. All prescription labels must include:

a. Trade name of the medication
b. Generic name of the medication
c. Address of the patient
d. Expiration date

36. How many milliliters of 95% alcohol should be mixed with 30% alcohol to make 2000 ml of a 40% alcohol solution?

a. 31
b. 108
c. 222
d. 308

37. How many grams of benzethonium chloride should be used in preparing 4 pints of a 1:1000 solution of benzethonium chloride?

a. 1.92
b. 3.86
c. 20
d. 38

38. How many milliequivalents of potassium gluconate are there in 2 tablespoonsful of a 30% potassium gluconate solution? (MW potassium gluconate = 234; valence = 1)

a. 21.65
b. 38.46
c. 390
d. 9000

39. The dose of a drug for a 150 lb. patient is 280 mg. How many milliliters of a product containing 180 mg/teaspoonful would provide the appropriate dose?

a. 4.9
b. 7.8
c. 12.7
d. 18.2

40. By law, patient package inserts must be provided to all patients receiving:

    a. A prescription medication for the first time only
    b. Certain prescription medications for the first time only
    c. Prescription medications in all instances, including refills
    d. Certain medications in all instances, including refills

41. The principle behind the use of the horizontal laminar airflow hood is:

    a. Air from the sterile compounding room is pumped directly through the hood horizontally to minimize contamination from microorganisms
    b. Filtered air flows from the hood toward the operator to provide a relatively clean work area
    c. Filtered air is provided in straight, parallel lines, flowing downward
    d. The operator is protected from the possible hazardous effects of cytotoxic agents

42. How many milliliters of a 0.5% sodium sulfate solution should be mixed with a 5% sodium sulfate solution to make a liter of 2% solution?

    a. 250
    b. 333
    c. 500
    d. 667

43. There are 18 grams of an expectorant in a liter of a cough syrup. How many grains of expectorant are contained in a teaspoonful dose of the cough syrup?

    a. 0.09
    b. 1.38
    c. 5.84
    d. 90

44. How many capsules each containing $1\frac{3}{8}$ gr. of a drug can be filled completely from a 28 g bottle of the drug?

    a. 24
    b. 32
    c. 313
    d. 431

45. If 4 fluid ounces of a solution cost $8.75, how much would a tablespoonful cost?

    a. $0.36
    b. $1.09
    c. $4.38
    d. $6.25

46. How many milliequivalents of potassium are in 2 g of potassium penicillin V if the molecular weight is 389 and the valence is 1?

    a. 5.14
    b. 78.2
    c. 154.6
    d. 389.3

47. What would be the infusion rate for a 50 mg/ml magnesium sulfate solution to provide 1.2 g/hr?

    a. 0.4 ml/min
    b. 2.5 ml/min
    c. 20 ml/min
    d. 24 ml/min

48. A 5 lb. 8 oz. neonate in the nursery requires 2.5 mg/kg of gentamicin. How many milliliters of solution containing 20 mg/ml should be administered?

    a. 0.029
    b. 0.31
    c. 2.5
    d. 6.3

49. A solution contains 5 mEq of calcium per 50 ml. How many milligrams of calcium would be contained in a liter of this solution? (AW calcium = 40; the valence = 2)

    a. 20
    b. 100
    c. 2000
    d. 4000

50. How many milligrams of benzocaine are needed to prepare the following prescription?

Rx	Glycerin	2.5%
	Benzocaine	2%
	Hydrophilic ung. qs	60 g

    a. 1.2
    b. 12
    c. 120
    d. 1200

51. How many grains of ephedrine are left in a 437.5 gr. bottle of ephedrine after compounding 400 capsules each containing $\frac{3}{8}$ gr. of ephedrine?

    a. 28.5
    b. 73.2
    c. 150.8
    d. 287.5

52. Which of the following is not a reliable factor to consider when identifying a manufacturing source for a particular drug?

    a. Purchase price
    b. Quantity of medication used by the pharmacy each year
    c. Policies that are used by other pharmacies for ordering their drug inventories
    d. Delivery turn-around time for orders

53. The instructions on a nafcillin vial say to add 3.4 ml of sterile water to the 1 g vial resulting in 4.1 ml of solution. How many milliliters would provide a 675 mg dose?

    a. 0.36
    b. 1.92
    c. 2.31
    d. 2.77

54. Assume in question #53 you accidentally used 4.3 ml of sterile water to reconstitute the 1 g vial of nafcillin. How many milliliters of this new solution would provide the 675 mg dose?

    a. 0.7
    b. 2.8
    c. 3.4
    d. 4.3

55. How many milliliters of a 0.1% solution can be made from 75 mg of a chemical

    a. 10 ml
    b. 75 ml
    c. 100 ml
    d. 750 ml

56. A compounded ointment requires it to be heated to 65°C. What would this reading be on a Fahrenheit thermometer?

    a. 18
    b. 68
    c. 149
    d. 172

57. Upon receipt, all of the following products should be stored under refrigeration except:

a. Insulin
b. Chlorpromazine concentrate
c. Mycostatin® pastilles
d. Famotidine injection

58. One gram of dextrose provides 3.4 calories. How many calories would be provided by a liter of a 50% dextrose solution?

a. 1.7
b. 17
c. 170
d. 1700

59. How many grams of coal tar are needed to compound 1 lb. of this prescription?

Rx

Coal Tar		2 g
Zinc Oxide Paste	qs	60 g

a. 2.3
b. 15.1
c. 16.2
d. 21.6

60. An intravenous solution containing 20,000 units of heparin in 500 ml of 0.45% sodium chloride solution is to be infused to provide 1000 units of heparin per hour. How many drops per minute should be infused to deliver the desired dose if the intravenous set calibrates at 15 gtts/ml?

a. 0.42
b. 6
c. 16
d. 32

61. How many colchicine tablets containing 600 mcg each can be prepared from 40 grams of colchicine?

a. 66
b. 666
c. 6,666
d. 66,666

62. How many grams of a 5% benzocaine ointment can be prepared by diluting 1 lb. of 20% benzocaine ointment with white petrolatum?

a. 129
b. 642
c. 735
d. 1,816

63. How many milligrams of pilocarpine nitrate are required to prepare 15 ml of an ophthalmic solution containing 0.25% pilocarpine nitrate?

a. 0.61
b. 18.2
c. 37.5
d. 380.9

64. How many 2.25 g sodium chloride tablets would be required to prepare 5 L of a 0.9% solution of sodium chloride?

a. 20
b. 70
c. 100
d. 2000

65. From the following formula, determine how many grams of calcium carbonate would be required to prepare 1 kg of the powder:

Magnesium oxide	1 part
Calcium carbonate	6 parts
Sodium bicarbonate	8 parts

a. 0.1
b. 30
c. 400
d. 750

66. Prochlorperazine injection is available in 10 ml multiple dose vials containing 5 mg/ml. How many 2.5 mg doses can be withdrawn from a single vial?

a. 4
b. 5
c. 20
d. 40

67. How many milliliters of water should be *added* to a quart of 10% boric acid solution to make a 3% solution?

    a. 1,120
    b. 1,600
    c. 2,240
    d. 3,200

Answers appear on pages 117–120.

Answer Key to Sample Questions

Chapter One

A. 4

B. 4

C.1. false

C.2. true

C.3. false
(if a patient requests a refill, the technician should notify the pharmacist)

D.1. no

D.2. yes

D.3. no

D.4. yes

D.5. no

D.6. no

D.7. yes

D.8. no

D.9. yes

D.10. yes

D.11. no

D.12. no

D.13. yes

D.14. no

D.15. yes

D.16. no

D.17. yes

E.1. Take two tablets by mouth four times a day.

E.2. Take one capsule before meals and at bedtime.

E.3. Inject 5 mg intramuscularly every 3–4 hours as needed for nausea.

E.4. Instill one drop into right eye every 12 hours.

E.5. Instill 2–3 drops into each ear three times a day.

E.6. Instill one drop into each ear twice daily.

F. 3

G. 5

Chapter Two

A.1. false

A.2. true

A.3. true

A.4. false

B. 5

Chapter Three

A.1. false

A.2. false

A.3. false

B. 2

C. 5

D.1. c

D.2. e

D.3. l

D.4. k

D.5. i

D.6. b

D.7. a

D.8. j

D.9. g

D.10. d

D.11. f

D.12. h

E. 5

F. 1

G. 3
(oral antineoplastic agents [e.g., tablets] should also be handled with caution but do not always require handling using aseptic technique or a vertical laminar airflow hood)

Chapter Four

A. 2

B.1. false

B.2. false

B.3. false
(some products, although slow moving, must be kept on hand)

C. 1

D.1. c

D.2. c

D.3. a

D.4. c

D.5. a

D.6. c

D.7. a

D.8. a

D.9. c

D.10. b

Chapter Five

A. 5

B. 1

Chapter Six

A.1. $\frac{10 \div 5}{75 \div 5} = \frac{2}{15}$

A.2. $\frac{8 \div 8}{16 \div 8} = \frac{1}{2}$

A.3. $\frac{3 \div 3}{15 \div 3} = \frac{1}{5}$

A.4. 60/186 = 30/93 = 10/31

B.1. 5 = 5/1

B.2. $3\frac{2}{3}$ = 11/3

C.1. 30/64, 12/64, 7/64

C.2. 18/24, 21/24, 10/24

D. 15/4 = $3\frac{3}{4}$

E. $3/4 + 1\frac{1}{8} = 6/8 + 9/8 = 15/8 = 1\frac{7}{8}$

F. $7\frac{5}{8} - 1\frac{1}{3} = 61/8 - 4/3 = 183/24 - 32/24 = 151/24 = 6\frac{7}{24}$

G. $1\frac{3}{4} \times 3 = 7/4 \times 3/1 = 21/4 = 5\frac{1}{4}$

H. $1/2 \div 5 = 1/2 \div 5/1 = 1/2 \times 1/5 = 1/10$

I. $3/16 \div 1\frac{1}{2} = 3/16 \div 3/2 = 3/16 \times 2/3 = 6/48 = 1/8$

J.1. 0.07 = 7/100

J.2. 0.077 = 77/1000

J.3. $5.0125 = 5\frac{125}{10,000} = 5\frac{1}{80}$

K.1. 3/8 = 0.375

K.2. $2\frac{7}{13}$ = 33/13 = 2.54

L.1. 3.75 – 1/2 = 3.75 – 0.5 = 3.25

L.2. 3/4 × 2.5 = 0.75 × 2.5 = 1.875

L.3. $2\frac{3}{8} \div 0.5 = 2.375 \div 0.5 = 4.75$

M.1. 29 = XXIX

M.2. 47 = XLVII

M.3. 86 = LXXXVI

M.4. 1154 = MCLIV

N.1. LXXVIII = 78

N.2. CXIII = 113

N.3. XCIV = 94

N.4. MCMLXI = 1961

O. 3/8 = 0.375
0.375 ÷ 0.0125 = 30 doses

P. Step 1: $2 \times 1.25 = 2.5$
$3 \times 1.75 = 5.25$
7.75 oz. dispensed
Step 2: $8 - 7.75 = 0.25$ oz. remaining in the bottle

Q. 1/200 ÷ 1/40 = 1/200 × 40/1 = 40/200 = 1/5 tablet

R. 1/150 ÷ 1/400 = 1/150 × 400/1 = 400/150 = $2\frac{2}{3}$

S. 10 × 44 = 440 = cdxl

Chapter Seven

A.1. 72% = 72/100 = 0.72

A.2. 0.35 = 35% = 35/100 = 7/20

A.3. 25% = 25/100 = 25:100

A.4. 0.182 = 18.2%

A.5. 3/8 = 0.375 = 37.5%

B.1. $40
A/B = C/D
10 lb./$200 = 2 lb./x
(x) (10 lb.) = ($200) (2 lb.)
$$x = \frac{(\$200)\ (2 \text{ lb.})}{10 \text{ lb.}}$$
x = $40

B.2. 1.25 lb.
A/B = C/D
10 lb./$25 = x/$25
($25) (10 lb.) = ($200) (x)
$$\frac{(\$25)\ (10 \text{ lb.})}{(\$200)} = x$$
1.25 lb = x

B.3. $12.50
Step 1: A/B = C/D
1 lb./16 oz. = 10 lb./x
$$\frac{(10 \text{ lb.})\ (16 \text{ oz.})}{1 \text{ lb.}} = x$$
x = 160 oz. (and this costs $200 as mentioned earlier)

Step 2: A/B = C/D
160 oz./$200 = 10 oz./x
(10 oz.) ($200) = (160 oz.) (x)
$$\frac{(10 \text{ oz.})\ (\$200)}{160 \text{ oz.}} = x$$
x = $12.50

C. 5.46 g
1000 tabs/11.5 g = 475 tabs/x
x = 5.46 g

D. 160 mg
5 mg/15 mls = x/480 ml
x = 160 mg

E. 32,500 mg
2 tabs/650 mg = 100 tabs/x
x = 32,500 mg

F. 300 tablets
7 tabs/35 mg = x/1500 mg
x = 300 tabs

G. $52.20
$0.58/1 tab = x/90 tabs
x = $52.20

H. 0.65 g
1 cap/0.0325 g = 20 caps/x
x = 0.65 g

I. $206.49
385 lb./$795 = 100 lb./x
x = $206.49

J. 78.64 kg
2.2 lb./1 kg = 173 lb./x
x = 78.64 kg

K. 300,000 units
6,000,000 units/10 ml = x/0.5 ml
x = 300,000 units

L. 300 ml
5 ml/1 min. = x/60 min.
x = 300 ml

M. 5,250 mg
750 mg/1 day = x/7 days
x = 5,250 mg

N. 11.2 mg
28 mg/3 ml = x/1.2 ml
x = 11.2 mg

O. 1.5 g
10 g/100 ml = x/15 ml
x = 1.5 g

P. $8.96
15 ml/$0.28 = 480 ml/x
x = $8.96

Chapter Eight

A.1. 225 km = 225,000 m
(1 km/1000 m = 225 km/x)

A.2. 525 g = 0.525 kg
(1 kg/1000 g = x/525 g)

A.3. 5 g = 5,000 mg
(1 g/1000 mg = 5 g/x)

5 g = 5,000,000 mcg
(1 g/1,000,000 mcg = 5 g/x)

A.4. 350 ml = 0.35 L
(1 L/1,000 ml = x/350 ml)

B.1. 60 gr.
(1 scr./20 gr. = 3 scr./x)

B.2. 24 scruples
(1 dram/3 scr. = 8 drams/x)

480 gr.
(1 dram/60 gr. = 8 drams/x)

B.3. 96 drams
(8 drams/1 oz. = x/12 oz.)
288 scruples
(3 scr./1 dram = x/96 drams)
5760 gr.
(1 scr./20 gr. = 288 scr./x)

B.4. 480 minims
(1 fluid dram/60 minims = 8 fluid drams/x)

B.5. 128 fluid drams
(8 fluid drams/1 fluid oz. = x/16 fluid oz.)

B.6. 32 fluid ounces
(1 pt/16 fluid oz. = 2 pt/x)

B.7. 8 pints
(2 pt/1 qt = x/4 qt)

128 fluid ounces
(16 oz./1 pt = x/8 pt)

C. 7000 gr.
(1 oz./437.5 gr. = 16 oz./x)

D. grain

E. none
(avoirdupois system only measures weight)

F. none
(must use conversion factors like 15.4 gr./gram and 30 ml/1 fl. oz.)

G.1. 0.065 grams
(1 g/15.4 gr. = x/1 gr.)

65 mg
(1 g/1000 mg = 0.065 g/x)

G.2. 437.5 gr.

28.4 grams
(1 g/15.4 gr. = x/437.5 gr.)

G.3. 16 oz.
454 grams
(1 oz./28.4 g = 16 oz./x)

7000 gr.
(1 g/15.4 gr. = 454 g/x)

0.454 kg
(1 kg/1000 g = x/454 g)

G.4. 480 gr.
31.1 grams
(1 g/15.4 gr. = x/480 gr.)

G.5. 2.2 lbs.
(454 g/1 lb. = 1000 g/x)

H.1. 16 fluid ounces
480 ml
(1 oz./30 ml = 16 oz./x)

H.2. 128 fluid ounces
(16 oz./1 pt = x/8 pt)

3840 ml
(1 oz./30 ml = 128 oz./x)

3.84 L
(1 L/1000 ml = x/3840 ml)

I. 68°F
°F = 32 + 9/5°C
°F = 32 + 9/5 (20)
°F = 32 + 36
°F = 68°

J. 100°C
°C = 5/9 (°F – 32)
°C = 5/9 (212 – 32)
°C = 5/9 (180)
°C = 100

K. 1,538 tablets
Step 1: 0.5 kg = 500 g = 500,000 mg
Step 2: 325 mg/1 tab = 500,000 mg/x
x = 1,538 tabs

L. 111.8 kg
2.2 lb./1 kg = 246 lb./x
x = 111.8 kg

M. 8,000 mcg
Step 1: 40 mg = 40,000 mcg
Step 2: 40,000 mcg/10 ml = x/2 ml
x = 8,000 mcg

N. 38.5 gr
Step 1: 10 g/1000 ml = x/250 ml
x = 2.5 g
Step 2: 1 g/15.4 gr. = 2.5 g/x
x = 38.5 gr.

Chapter Nine

A.1. 3 tsp.
(1 tsp./5 ml = x/15 ml)

A.2. 6 tsp.
(1 tsp./5 ml = x/30 ml)

2 tbsp.
(1 tbsp./15 ml = x/30 ml)

A.3. 16 fluid ounces
480 ml
(1 fluid oz./30 ml = 16 fluid oz./x)

32 tbsp.
(1 tbsp./15 ml = x/480 ml)

96 tsp.
(1 tbsp./3 tsp. = 32 tbsp./x)
or
(1 tsp./5 ml = x/480 ml)

B.1. 2.2 lb.
(454 g/1 lb. = 1000 g/x)

B.2. 0.4 g
(20 mg/2.2 lb. = x/44 lb.)
x = 400 mg = 0.4 g

B.3. 133 mg
(400 mg/3 doses = 133 mg/1 dose)

B.4. approximately 1
(125 mg/1 tsp. = 133 mg/x)
x = 1.064 tsp.

B.5. approximately 3
(125 mg/1 tsp. = 400 mg/x)
x = 3.2 tsp.

B.6. 150 ml
(15 ml/1 day = x/10 days)

B.7. 5 fluid ounces
(1 fluid oz./30 ml = x/150 ml)

B.8. 21 doses
(3 doses/1 day = x/7 days)

C. 180 ml
Step 1: (15 ml/1 dose = x/4 doses)
x = 60 ml/day
Step 2: (60 ml/1 day = x/3 days)
x = 180 ml

D.1. 600 ml
Step 1: (30 drops/1 min. = x/360 min.)
x = 10,800 drops
Step 2: (18 drops/1 ml = 10,800 drops/x)
x = 600 ml

D.2. 5.4 grams
(0.9 g NaCl/100 ml = x/600 ml)

E.1. 4.3 minutes
Step 1: (1 kg/2.2 lb. = 90 kg/x)
x = 198 lb.

Step 2: (1 mcg/1 lb. = x/198 lb.)
x = 198 mcg = 0.198 mg/min.
Step 3: (0.198 mg/1 min. = 0.85 mg/x)

x = 4.3 min.

E.2. 0.5 ml/min.
(2 mg/5 ml = 0.198 mg/x)

E.3. 2.15 ml
(0.5 ml/1 min. = x/4.3 min.)
or
(2 mg/5 ml = 0.85 mg/x)
x = 2.13 ml

F. 3.33 ml
Step 1: (6 mg/lb. = x/50 lb.)
x = 300 mg

Step 2: (90 mg/1 ml = 300 mg/x)
x = 3.33 ml

G. 120 tablets
Step 1: (5 mg/lb. = x/100 lb.)
x = 500 mg daily

Step 2: (125 mg/tab = 500 mg/x)
x = 4 tabs daily

Step 3: (4 tabs/day = x/30 days)
x = 120 tabs

H. 2.4 ml
Step 1: (1 kg/2.2 lb. = x/66 lb.)
x = 30 kg patient's weight

Step 2: (10 mg/1 kg = x/30 kg)
x = 300 mg

Step 3: (125 mg/1 ml = 300 mg/x)
x = 2.4 ml

I. 0.4 ml
Step 1: 100 mcg = 0.1 mg
Step 2: (0.5 mg/2 ml = 0.1 mg/x)
x = 0.4 ml

J. 0.59 mg
Step 1: (28 gtts/1 ml = 15 gtts/x)
x = 0.54 ml
Step 2: (1.1 mg/1 ml = x/0.54 ml)
x = 0.59 mg

Chapter Ten

A.1. 19.2 g
(5 g trieth/1000 ml = x/3,840 ml)
x = 19.2 g = 19,200 mg
(1 g/1000 mg = 19.2 g/x)

A.2. 148 gr.
Step 1: (20 g/1000 ml = x/480 ml)
x = 9.6 g
Step 2: (1 g/15.4 gr. = 9.6 g/x)
x = 148 gr.

A.3. 5 tsp.
Step 1: (250 ml B.B./1000 ml lotion = x/100 ml lotion)
x = 25 ml B.B.
Step 2: (1 tsp./5 ml = x/25 ml)
x = 5 tsp.

B. 1.67%
(2 g/120 g = 0.0167 = 1.67%)

B.1. 16.7 mg
2 g sulfur/120 g.ung = x/1 g.ung
x = 0.0167 g = 16.7 mg

C. 4.4%
(20 g/454 g = 0.044 = 4.4%)

D. 29.4%
50 g/(50 g + 120 g) = 0.294 = 29.4%
Note: The 50 g sulfur was added to 120 g petrolatum, so the final product weighed 170 g

D.1. 70.6%
(120 g pet./170 g.ung = 0.706 = 70.6%)
Note: could also take previous answer and subtract from 100%, i.e., 100% – 29.4% = 70.6%

E. 22.5 g ZnO
(0.25 × 90 g = 22.5 g)

F. 6.25%
(30 ml/480 ml = 0.0625 = 6.25%)

F.1. 3.75 ml
(30 ml/480 ml = x/60 ml)
or
(0.0625 × 60 = 3.75 ml)

G. 4.67%
(7 g/150 ml = 0.0467 = 4.67%)

H. 11.8%
(454 g/3840 ml = 0.118 = 11.8%)

H.1. 1:8.46
454 g/3840 ml = 1/x
x = 8.46
the ratio is 1/8.46 or 1:8.46

I. 48 g
(0.10 × 480 = 48)

I.1. 10%
(percent is the same for any volume of a percent solution)

J. 2%
(1:50 = 1/50 = 0.02 = 2%)

19.2 g
(0.02 × 960 ml = 19.2 g)

K. 60 mg
Step 1: (6% means 6 g/100 ml) or 6000 mg/100 ml
Step 2: (6000 mg/100 ml = x/1 ml)

K.1. 1:16.67
6% = 6 g/100 ml
6 g/100 ml = 1/x
x = 16.67
the ratio is 1/16.67 or 1:16.67

L. 0.83%
Step 1: (2000 mg = 2 g) and (8 fluid ounces = 240 ml)
Step 2: (2 g/240 ml = 0.0083 = 0.83%)

1:120
(2 g/240 ml = 1/x x = 120)

8.33 mg
(2000 mg/240 ml = x/1 ml)

M. 1:120
(6/720 = 1/x x = 120)
(so 6:720 equals 1:120)

M.1. 0.833%
6/720 = 0.00833 = 0.833%

N. 1.063%
[(30 ml) (17%) = (480 ml) (x)]

N.1. 1:94
(1.063/100 = 1/x x = 94)

N.2. 10.63 mg
Step 1: 1.063 g/100 ml = 1063 mg/100 ml

Step 2: (1063 mg/100 ml = x/1 ml) x = 10.63 mg

N.3. 0.85 g
(0.17 × 5 ml = 0.85)

N.4. 4.25%
[(5 ml) (17%) = (20 ml) (x)]
x = 4.25%

Note: The final solution is 20 ml (5 ml added to 15 ml)

N.5. 78.54 gr.
Step 1: 0.17 × 30 = 5.1 g

Step 2: 1 g/15.4 gr. = 5.1 g/x
x = 78.54 gr.

N.6. 78.54 gr.
The benzalkonium chloride in the initial 30 ml is all that will be in the final 480 ml. The 30 ml was diluted with a diluent that does not contain any additional benzalkonium chloride

N.7. 1:2000
[(100 ml) (0.5%) = (1000 ml) (x)]
x = 0.05% = 0.0005 = 5/10,000 = 5:10,000 = 1:2000

N.8. 2.5 mg
Step 1: 5 g/10,000 ml
5000 mg/10,000 ml

Step 2: 5000 mg/10,000 ml = x/5 ml
or
0.0005 (5 ml) = 0.0025 g = 2.5 mg

O. yes
(10% is between 5% and 20%)

O.1. 151 g of 20%
(Alligation Alternate)
Note: The total amount made of 10% is the sum of the parts (5 parts + 10 parts = 15 parts). In this case, it is 454 grams, so

$$\frac{15\ parts}{454\ g} = \frac{5\ parts}{x}$$

303 g of 5%
(15 parts/454 = 10 parts/x)
or
(454 g (total) – 151 g (of 20%) = 303 g of 5%)

O.2. 90 g of 10%
(5 parts/30 g = 15 parts/x)

P. no
(10% is not between 20% and 15%)

P.1. not possible

P.2. not possible

Q. 9 g NaCl

(0.009 × 1000 ml = 9 g)

153.8 mEq Na^+
58.5 mg/1 mEq = 9000 mg/x
Note: MW of NaCl = 58.5

R. 0.745%
Step 1: MW KCl = 74.5 mg = 1 mEq

Step 2: 10 mEq = 745 mg = 0.745 g

Step 3: 0.745 g/100 ml = 0.00745 = 0.745%

R.1. 7,450 mg
Step 1: 10 mEq/100 ml = x/1000 ml
x = 100 mEq

Step 2: 1 mEq KCl/74.5 mg KCl = 100 mEq KCl/x
x = 7,450 mg

S. 4.5 mEq
Step 1: mEq $CaCl_2$ = 111/2 = 55.5 mg

Step 2: 55.5 mg/1 mEq = 250 mg/x

T. 1.67%
Step 1: 250 mg = 0.25 g

Step 2: 0.25 g/15 ml = 0.0167 = 1.67%

U. 38.5 mEq
Step 1: MW of $Al(OH)_3$ = 78
Step 2: 1 mEq = 78/3 = 26 mg
Step 3: 1 mEq $Al(OH)_3$/26 mg = x/1000 mg

V.1. 200 ml
(5 ml/dose × 4 doses/day × 10 days = 200 ml)

V.2. 40 ml
(200 ml – 160 ml H_2O = 40 ml)

V.3. 7 g
(1 gram/1 day = x/7 days)

W. 8.33 tablets
Step 1: (1 cap/5 mg codeine = 50 caps/x)
x = 250 mg
Step 2: (30 mg/1 tab = 250 mg/x)

X. 12 tablets
Step 1: (0.02 × 150) = 3 g = 3000 mg)
Step 2: (250 mg/1 tab = 3000 mg/x)
x = 12 tabs

X.1. 1:50
Note: 1 teaspoonful of 2% is still 2%, so 2% = 0.02 = 2/100 = 2:100 = 1:50

X.2. 20 mg
Step 1: 2% × 150 = 3 g = 3,000 mg
Step 2: 3000 mg/150 ml = x/1 ml
x = 20 mg

Y.1. 7500 mg

$$\frac{500\ mg}{1\ ml} = \frac{x}{15\ ml}$$

Y.2. no

Y.3. yes

Y.4. 2.2 ml
15 ml (final volume) – 12.8 ml (diluent) = 2.2 ml (powder volume displacement)

Y.5. 4 ml

$$\frac{500\ mg}{1\ ml} = \frac{2000\ mg}{x}$$

Y.6. 3.25 ml
10 ml (diluent) + 2.2 ml (powder volume displacement) = 12.2 ml (final volume containing 7500 mg of the drug)

$$\frac{7500\ mg}{12.2\ ml} = \frac{2000\ mg}{x}$$

Z. 8.25%
Use Alligation Medial Method
0.5 kg × 3% = 1.5 kg%
1.5 kg × 10% = 15.0 kg%
2.0 kg 16.5 kg%

16.5 kg%/2 kg = 8.25%

Z.1. 1:12.12
(8.25/100 = 1/x) x = 12.12

Z.2. 37.5 g
454 × 8.25% = 37.5 g

Z.3. no

Z.4. 237.8 g
Use Alligation Alternate
Step 1:

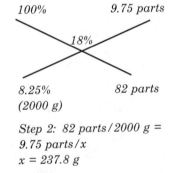

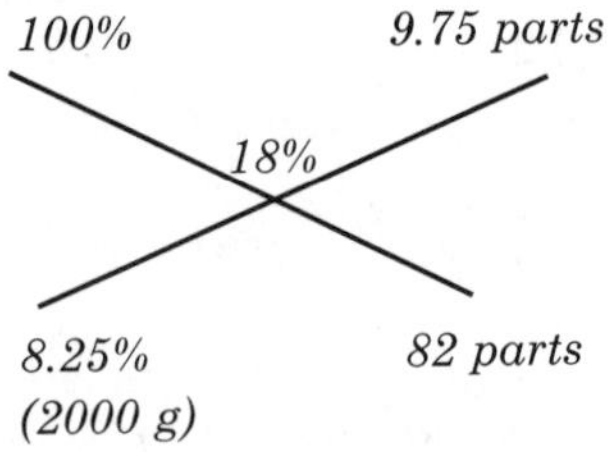

Step 2: 82 parts/2000 g = 9.75 parts/x
x = 237.8 g

Chapter Eleven

A. $20
(1 capsule/$0.20 = 100 capsules/x)

A.1. $0.25 each
($0.20 cost plus $0.05 profit)

A.2. $7.50

$$\frac{1\ cap}{\$0.25} = \frac{30\ caps}{x}$$

B.1. $10
selling price = cost + markup
$60 = $50 + markup
markup = $60 – $50 = $10

B.2. 20%
$\frac{markup}{cost} = \frac{\$10}{\$50} = 0.2 = 20\%$

B.3. 16.7%
$\frac{markup}{selling\ price} = \frac{\$10}{\$60} =$
0.167 = 16.7%

Chapter Twelve

1. c

2. d
1 g/30,000 ml = x/3000
x = 0.1 g = 100 mg

3. b
Step 1: 250 units/1 g = x/1000 g
x = 250,000 units

Step 2: 500 units/1 g = 250,000 units/x   x = 500 g

4. c

5. a
Step 1: 10,000 mcg = 10 mg = 0.01 g

Step 2: 0.1 g/10 ml = 0.01 g/x
x = 1 ml

6. d
0.25% × 30 = 0.0025 × 30 = 0.075 g = 75 mg

7. c

8. c
Step 1: 30 mEq/1000 ml = 5 mEq/x
x = 167 ml

Step 2: 167 ml/60 minutes = x/1 minute
x = 2.78 ml per minute

Step 3: 15 gtts/1 ml = x/2.78 ml
x = 41.7 or 42 gtts/min

9. a
0.9 g/100 ml = 60 g/x
x = 6,666 ml = 6.67 liters

10. d
Step 1: Use Alligation Alternate

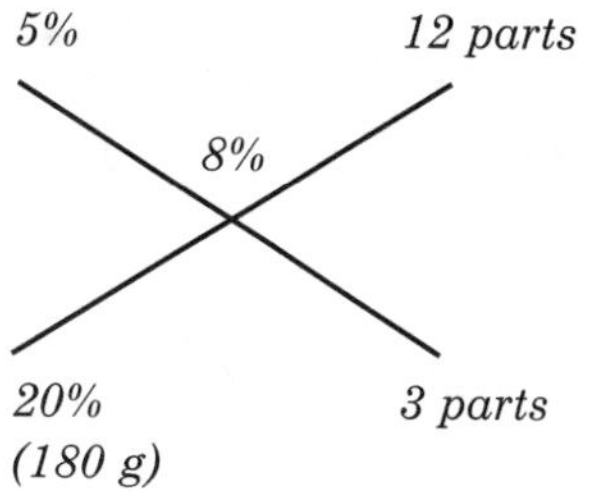

Step 2: 3 parts/180 g = 12 parts/x
x = 720 g

11. b
2000 mg/5.8 ml = x/1 ml
x = 345 mg

12. d

13. b

14. a
Step 1: 2.2 lb./1 kg = 220 lb./x
x = 100 kg

Step 2: 5 mcg/1 kg = x/100 kg
x = 500 μg = 0.5 mg per min

Step 3: 0.5 mg/1 min = x/60 min
x = 30 mg per hour

Step 4: 800 mg/500 ml = 30 mg/x
x = 18.75 ml

(Note: Sometimes μg is used to represent micrograms or mcg)

15. c
Step 1: 2.2 lb./1 kg = 264 lb./x
x = 120 kg

Step 2: 10 mg/1 kg = x/120 kg
x = 1200 mg

Step 3: 200 mg/1 tab = 1200 mg/x
x = 6 tabs

16. c
1 g/750 ml = x/960 ml
x = 1.28 g

17. c

18. a
Step 1: total weight of recipe
400 + 150 + 100 + 350 = 1000 g

Step 2: 400 g glycerin/1000 g zinc gel. = x/454 g zinc gel
x = 181.6 g

19. a

20. b
Step 1: ½ pint = 240 ml
Step 2: 2 gal = 7,680 ml
Step 3: 1 bottle/240 ml = x/7,680 ml
x = 32 bottles

21. b

22. b
Step 1: Alligation Medial
90 ml × 14% = 1260 ml%
100 ml × 0% = 0
40 ml × 78% = 3120 ml%
230 ml 4380 ml%
Step 2: 4380 ml%/230 ml = 19.04%

23. c

24. c
Step 1: 2.2 lb./1 kg = 38 lb./x
x = 17.27 kg
Step 2: 35 mg/1 kg = x/17.27 kg
x = 604.54 mg (total daily dose)
Step 3: 604.54 mg/6 doses = x/1 dose
x = 100.8 mg per dose

25. d
0.5 mg/2 ml = x/0.75 ml
x = 0.1875 mg = 187.5 mcg

26. a

27. a
Step 1: 1 mEq = 74.5 mg/1 (valence) = 74.5 mg
Step 2: 74.5 mg/1 mEq = x/3 mEq
x = 223.5 mg
Step 3: 223.5 mg/5 ml = x/1000 ml
x = 44,700 mg = 44.7 g

28. a
(old vol)(old %) = (new vol)(new %)
(x) (20%) = (600 ml) (0.5%)
x = 15 ml

29. b

30. b
Step 1: Alligation Alternate

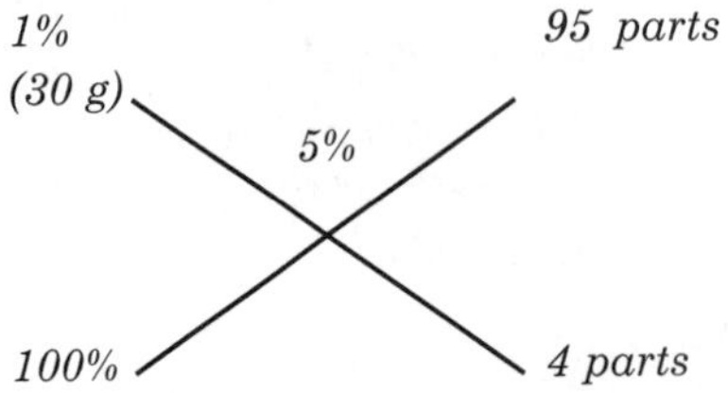

Step 2: 95 parts/30 g = 4 parts/x
x = 1.26 g

31. c
500 mcg/15 ml = x/1000 ml
x = 33,333 mcg = 33.33 mg

32. c
3 g/$24.50 = 0.5 g/x x = $4.08

33. d
Step 1: 500 mg/1 dose = x/4 doses
x = 2000 mg per day
Step 2: 2000 mg/1 day = x/10 days
x = 20,000 mg for 10 days
Step 3: 250 mg/5 ml = 20,000 mg/x
x = 400 ml

34. c

35. d

36. d
Step 1: Alligation Alternate

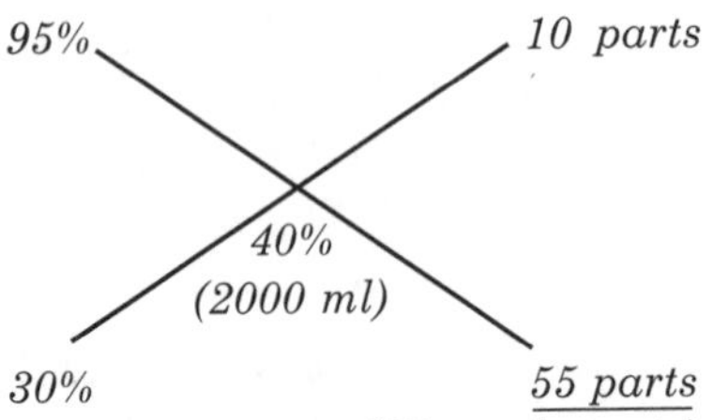

(65 total parts)

Step 2: 65 parts/2000 ml = 10 parts/x
x = 308 ml

37. a
Step 1: 4 × 480 ml = 1920 ml
Step 2: 1 g/1000 ml = x/1920 ml
x = 1.92 g

38. b
Step 1: 1 mEq potassium gluconate = MW/valence = 234/1 = 234 mg
Step 2: 2 tablespoonsful = 30 ml
Step 3: 30 ml × 30% = 9 g
(i.e., 30 ml × 0.3 = 9 g)
Step 4: 9 g = 9,000 mg
Step 5: 1 mEq K. gluconate/234 mg = x/9,000 mg
x = 38.46 mEq

39. b
180 mg/5 ml = 280 mg/x
x = 7.78 ml

40. d
(Examples include: oral contraceptives, products containing estrogenic or progestational agents, isotretinoin, intrauterine devices, and isoproterenol inhalation devices.)

41. b

42. d
Step 1: Alligation Alternate

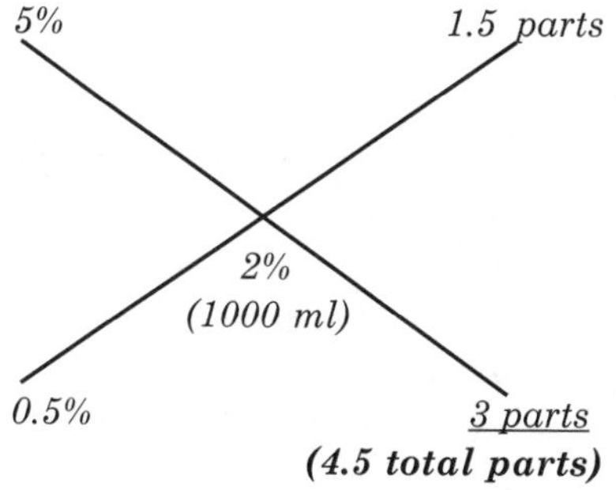

Step 2: 4.5 parts/1000 ml = 3 parts/x
x = 667 ml

43. b
Step 1: 18 g/1000 ml = x/5 ml
x = 0.09 g = 90 mg
Step 2: 65 mg/1 gr. = 90 mg/x
x = 1.38 gr

44. c
Step 1: 1 g/15.4 gr. = 28 g/x
x = 431.2 gr.
Step 2: $1\frac{3}{8}$ *gr./1 capsule = 431.2 gr./x*
x = 313 capsules

45. b
$8.75/120 ml = x/15 ml
x = $1.09

46. a
Step 1: 1 mEq = MW/valence = 389/1 = 389 mg
Step 2: 1 mEq K. Pcn.V/389 mg = x/2000 mg
x = 5.14 mEq

47. a
Step 1: 1200 mg/60 min = x/1 min
x = 20 mg per minute
Step 2: 50 mg/1 ml = 20 mg/x
x = 0.4 ml

48. b
Step 1: 2.2 lb./1 kg = 5.5 lb./x
x = 2.5 kg (infant's weight)
Step 2: 2.5 mg gentamicin/1 kg = x/2.5 kg
x = 6.25 mg (dose)
Step 3: 20 mg gentamicin/1 ml = 6.25 mg gentamicin/x
x = 0.31 ml

49. c
Step 1: 1 mEq calcium = AW/valence = 40/2 = 20 mg
Step 2: 1 mEq/20 mg = 5 mEq/x
x = 100 mg
Step 3: 100 mg/50 ml = x/1000 ml
x = 2000 mg per liter

50. d
2% × 60 g = 1.2 g = 1,200 mg benzocaine
(i.e., 0.02 × 60 = 1.2)

51. d
Step 1: 400 gr. × 3/8 = 150 gr.
Step 2: 437.5 gr. – 150 gr. = 287.5 gr.

52. c

53. d
1000 mg/4.1 ml = 675 mg/x
x = 2.77 ml

54. c
Step 1: From problem #53 the dry powder displacement is 0.7 ml
4.1 – 3.4 = 0.7 ml
Step 2: For problem #54
4.3 ml + 0.7 ml = 5 ml
(new and incorrect volume)
Step 3: Note: the 5 ml contains 1 g of nafcillin
1000 mg/5 ml = 675 mg/x
x = 3.375 = 3.4 ml

55. b
Step 1: 0.1% = 0.1 g/100 ml = 100 mg/100 ml
Step 2: 100 mg/100 ml = 75 mg/x
x = 75 ml

56. c
°F = 32 + 9/5°C
°F = 32 + (9/5 × 65)
°F = 32 + 117
°F = 149

57. b

58. d
Step 1: 50% = 50 g/100 ml
Step 2: 50 g/100 ml = x/1000 ml
x = 500 g
Step 3: 1 g dextrose/3.4 calories = 500 g dextrose/x
x = 1,700 calories

59. b

2 g coal tar/60 g formula = x/454 g formula
x = 15.1 g coal tar

60. b

Step 1: 1000 units/60 min = x/1 min
x = 16.67 units per minute

Step 2: 20,000 units/500 ml = 16.67 units/x
x = 0.42 ml per min

Step 3: 15 gtts/1 ml = x/0.42 ml
x = 6.3 gtts = 6 gtts/min

61. d

Step 1: 40 g = 40,000 mg = 40,000,000 mcg

Step 2: 600 μg/1 tablet = 40,000,000 μg/x
x = 66,666 tablets

62. d

Note: Since the diluent is ***zero*** *percent, this problem can be worked several ways. The easiest method is by a simple dilution, i.e., (old volume)(old %) = (new volume)(new %). A second method is alligation alternate, but this requires additional work.*

(O.V.) (O.%) = (N.V.) (N.%)
(454 g) (20%) = (x) (5%)
x = 1,816 g of 5%

63. c

Step 1: 0.25% = 0.25 g/100 ml = 250 mg/100 ml

Step 2: 250 mg/100 ml = x/15 ml
x = 37.5 mg

or

0.25% × 15 ml = 0.0375 g = 37.5 mg

64. a

Step 1: 5000 ml × 0.9% = 5,000 × 0.009 = 45 g

Step 2: 2.25 g/1 tablet = 45 g/x
x = 20 tablets

65. c

Step 1: Total parts in this formula equal 15
1 + 6 + 8 = 15 parts

Step 2: 15 parts powder/1000 g = 6 parts/x
x = 400 g of calcium carbonate

66. c

Step 1: 5 mg/1 ml = 2.5 mg/x
x = 0.5 ml per dose

Step 2: 0.5 ml/1 dose = 10 ml/x
x = 20 doses

67. c

Note: diluent is ***zero*** *percent so this can be solved by 2 methods.*

Step 1: (O.V.) (O.%) = (N.V.) (N.%)
(960 ml) (10%) = (x) (3%)
x = 3,200 ml of 3% dilution made, but how much water must be added to the 960 ml?

Step 2: 3,200 ml – 960 ml = 2,240 ml of water added

or

Step 1: Alligation Alternate

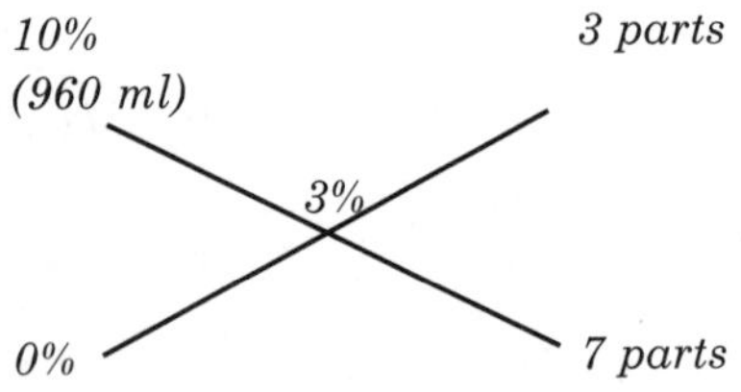

Step 2: 3 parts/960 ml = 7 parts/x
x = 2,240 ml water

Appendix A

Common Dosage Forms

aerosol
capsule
cream
drops
elixir

emulsion
enema
extract
gel
granule
injection
lotion

lozenge
ointment
paste
patch
pellet or implant
powder
solution
suppository
suspension
syrup
tablet
tincture

Drug Administration Routes

buccal
epidural
inhalation
intra-arterial
intracardiac
intramuscular
intranasal
intraperitoneal
intrathecal
intravenous
nasal
ophthalmic

oral
otic
parenteral
perivascular
rectal
subcutaneous
sublingual
topical
transdermal
urethral
urogenital
vaginal

Appendix B

Common Abbreviations Used in Prescriptions/Medication Orders

a	before
a.a. or aa	of each
a.c.	before meals
ad	up to
a.d.	right ear
ad lib.	at pleasure
a.m.	morning
ante	before
aq.	aqueous (water)
a.s.	left ear
a.u.	each ear
b.i.d.	twice a day
c. or c	with
cap.	capsule
cc.	cubic centimeter (milliliter)
Cl	chloride
comp.	compound
D.A.W.	dispense as written
D.C., dc, or disc.	discontinue
dil.	dilute
disp.	dispense
div.	divide
d.t.d.	give of such doses
dx	diagnosis
D5NS	5% dextrose in 0.9% sodium chloride
D5RL	5% dextrose in Ringer's lactate
D5W	5% dextrose in water
elix.	elixir
et	and
ex. aq.	in water
ft.	make
g or gm or Gm	gram
gal.	gallon
GI	gastrointestinal
gr.	grain
gtt.	drop
h. or hr.	hour
h.s.	at bedtime
hx	history
H_2O	water
IM	intramuscular
inj.	injection
IV	intravenous
IVP	intravenous push
IVPB	intravenous piggyback
K	potassium
KCl	potassium chloride
L or l	liter
lb.	pound
LR	lactated Ringer's
mcg or μg	microgram
mEq	milliequivalent
Mg	magnesium
mg	milligram
ml	milliliter
Na	sodium
NaCl	sodium chloride
N.F.	National Formulary
noct.	night
non rep.	do not repeat
NPO	nothing by mouth
NS	normal saline (0.9% sodium chloride)
NTG	nitroglycerin
N/V	nausea and/or vomiting
o.d.	right eye
o.l. or o.s	left eye
o.u.	both eyes
oz.	ounce
p̄	after
p.c.	after meals
p.m.	afternoon; evening
p.o.	by mouth
pr	per rectum
p.r.n.	as needed
pt.	pint
pulv.	powder
q.	every
q.d.	every day
q.h.	every hour
q.h.s.	every bedtime
q.i.d.	four times a day

q.o.d.	every other day
q.s.	a sufficient quantity
q.s. ad	a sufficient quantity to make
RL	Ringer's lactate
R/O	rule out
rt., R	right
s. or $\bar{s}$	without
Sig.	write on label
SL, sl	sublingual
sol.	solution
ss. or $\bar{s}\bar{s}$	one half
SSKI	saturated solution of potassium iodide
stat	immediately
s.c. or s.q.	subcutaneously
supp.	suppository
susp.	suspension
syr.	syrup
tab.	tablet
tbsp. or T	tablespoonsful
t.i.d.	three times a day
TPN	total parenteral nutrition
tr. or tinct.	tincture
tsp. or t.	teaspoonsful
u.d.	as directed
ung.	ointment
U.S.P.	United States Pharmacopoeia

Appendix C

Suggested Reading

American Society of Health-System Pharmacists. Manual for Pharmacy Technicians, second edition. Bethesda, MD: American Society of Health-System Pharmacists; 1998.

American Society of Health-System Pharmacists. Pharmacy Technician Certification Review and Practice Exam. Bethesda, MD: American Society of Health-System Pharmacists; 1998.

Ballington DA, Laughlin MM. Pharmacology for Technicians. St. Paul: EMC Paradigm; 1999.

Ballington DA, Laughlin MM. Pharmacology for Technicians Workbook. St. Paul: EMC Paradigm; 1999.

Ballington DA, Laughlin MM. Pharmacy Math for Technicians. St. Paul: EMC Paradigm; 1999.

Ballington DA. Pharmacy Practice for Technicians. St. Paul: EMC Paradigm; 1999.

Buerki RA, Vottero LD. Ethical Practices in Pharmacy: A Guidebook for Pharmacy Technicians. Madison, WI: American Institute of the History of Pharmacy; 1997.

Covington, TR, ed. Handbook of Nonprescription Drugs, 11th edition. Washington, DC: American Pharmaceutical Association; 1996.

Drug Facts and Comparisons. St. Louis: Facts and Comparisons; 1999.

Durgin JM, Hanan ZI, Mastanduono J, eds. Pharmacy Practice for Technicians, second edition. Albany: Delmar Publishers; 1999.

Harteker LR. The Pharmacy Technician Companion: Your Road Map to Technician Training and Careers. Washington, DC: American Pharmaceutical Association; 1998.

Kocher K. Pharmacy Certified Technician Calculations Workbook. Lansing, MI: Michigan Pharmacists Association; 1994.

Lance LL, Lacy C, Goldman MP. Drug Information Handbook for the Allied Health Professional, sixth edition. Hudson, OH: Lexi-Comp; 1999.

McEvoy GK, ed. AHFS Drug Information 1999. Bethesda, MD: American Society of Health-System Pharmacists; 1999.

The Pharmacy Technician. Englewood, CO: Morton Publishing Company; 1999.

Pharmacy Technician Review Series [workbook and video]. Waverly, IA: Pharmacy Marketing Group; 1998.

Pharmacy Technician Workbook and Certification Review. Englewood, CO: Morton Publishing Company; 1999.

Schumann W, Vander Linde JB. Pharmacy Certified Technician Training Manual, seventh edition. Lansing, MI: Michigan Pharmacists Association; 1997.

Stanaszek WF, Stanaszek MJ, Holt RJ, Strauss S. Understanding Medical Terms: A Guide for Pharmacy Practice, second edition. Lancaster, PA: Technomic Publishing Company; 1998.

Stoklosa MJ, Ansel HC. Pharmaceutical Calculations, 10th edition. Philadelphia: Lippincott Williams & Wilkins; 1995.

Strauss S. Strauss's Federal Drug Laws and Examination Review, fifth edition. Lancaster, PA: Technomic Publishing Company; 1997.